TAMING AUTISM

TAMING
AUTISM

REWIRING the BRAIN to RELIEVE SYMPTOMS
and SAVE LIVES

CHERYL L. NYE

PSYCHOLOGIST

ISBN 978-1-7353577-1-3

Library of Congress Control Number 2020912273

Publisher's Cataloging-in-Publication Data

Names: Nye, Cheryl L., author

Title: Taming autism: rewiring the brain to relieve symptoms and save lives / Cheryl L. Nye

Description: Lincoln University, PA: Child Stress Center, 2020.

Identifiers: LCCN 2020912273 (print) | ISBN 978-1-7353577-1-3 (paperback) | ISBN 978-1-7353577-0-6 (ebook)Subjects: LCSH: Autism-Treatment. | Autism-Psychological aspects. | Stress (psychology) | Mindfulness (Psychology) | BISAC: PSYCHOLOGY / PSYCHOPATHOLOGY / Autism Spectrum Disorders.

Classification: LCC RC553.A88 N94 2020 (print) | LCC RC553.A88 (ebook) | DDC 616.85/882-dc23.

To Ted Nawalinski and my husband, David Lopez, for always being there.

CONTENTS

INTRODUCTION

Revolutionary findings from the fields of neuroscience and psychology blend seamlessly to provide evidence of the harm caused by stress. Excessive stress damages brain neuroarchitecture and alters genes. The ability to regulate stress is compromised in those with autism and, as a result, excessive stress hormones cause and exacerbate their symptoms. Stress likely contributes to their shorter life spans. While researchers scramble to determine the elusive cause of autism, stress associated with this disorder runs rampant. Stress is often overlooked and underestimated due to its curious nature in autism. When addressed, interventions are frequently ineffective and potentially harmful. These include prescription drugs and ill-conceived behavioral strategies. When stress is safely and effectively treated, symptoms improve, symptoms that conceivably might also have been prevented. The foundation for this book is based upon empirical research from across the globe published in peer-reviewed journals with contributions from many disciplines. The book emerged following a unique professional experiment. My work progressed by compiling findings for nearly a decade generated in clinics and laboratories that now need to be translated for practical application to schools and homes. This book is a call to action for "Taming Autism."

DISCLAIMER

As a precaution, all are advised to check with their family physician before following any advice or beginning any program recommended in this book. Preliminary findings indicate the programs are safe and effective, but medical advice should be sought in advance of any proposed treatment.

PART I

WHAT IN THE WORLD IS GOING ON?

Chapter 1
WHAT HAPPENED?

It was at the close of the fourth session when my life changed. A boy who stood shoulder height and whose head was covered with dusty brown hair tugged at my elbow. He looked up and said, "Lady, when I do tai chi I don't feel crazy." His crystal-blue eyes locked with mine and I knew something remarkable had just happened. I was baffled and could make no sense of this child's proclamation. As a psychologist I take pride in unscrambling messages by reading facial expressions, inspecting context clues, and searching for motives, but I was flabbergasted. What on Earth had he just experienced? Why had he felt compelled to share this unsolicited comment? His words uprooted my professional career and set it on a new path for the next decade. It was on a lark that I began the practice of tai chi. My daughter had set off for college leaving a stark, empty nest behind. Despondent, I relied upon my own professional advice and took matters in hand. I searched for a new venture to help fill the void. To broaden my horizons, I enrolled in a tai chi class at the neighborhood YMCA. I was clueless about tai chi, but soon learned it was originally a martial art that had transformed into a meditative practice for tranquility. Tai chi consists of slow deliberate movements typically performed by a group of people who are silent during the routines. Even though I stumbled awkwardly in the initial sessions, I felt stuck since I had previously made a commitment to never quit anything again just because it was too difficult. As I acquired the routines, I began to perceive unexpected changes. I do not recall any specific incident but my ability to plan and organize improved. My "executive functioning" was considerably better. I started showing up on time. I planned and accomplished tasks prior to the last minute like putting gasoline in my car before the warning lights blinked. Others close to me remarked at the differences. It made no sense. I speculated whether those with ADHD who have notoriously poor executive functions might also improve.

With the assistance of school administrators at a local elementary school, I initiated a trial program for children with special needs. The group was formed to practice tai chi and consisted of young elementary school boys diagnosed with ADHD, autism, and Tourette syndrome. The administration granted permission with the caveat that the parents had to provide their own transportation and arrive an hour earlier than usual prior to the start of the school day. I was hopeful, but skeptical of the potential for success, especially with the additional inconvenience to the parents.

My fears escalated as the starting date approached. How could active, easily distracted, and impulsive young boys cooperate in such a slow-moving quiet exercise? How could they possibly remain engaged for a one-hour session? What was I thinking? I prepared obsessively. I drew on every bit of knowledge from my past experiences as a psychologist working with youth that I could recollect. I designed a program using educational strategies formulated on learning theories hammered into me in graduate school. Keep the exercises short. Change exercises. Reinforce frequently. Use a variety of reinforcers. My pockets were full with stickers and poker chips for my token economy. Exercises were carefully chosen and rehearsed. Unexpectedly, the boys took to the practice like the proverbial ducks to water. The weeks progressed, and they grew more adept and engaged over time in the exercise routines. Attendance rates remained over 90%.

My enthusiasm, however, waned. Near the end of the scheduled sessions I had grown bored and reluctant to even bother meeting with the parents again. My curiosity regarding the "I don't feel crazy" comment was fading, but I dutifully recalled the parents and dredged on. Unexpectedly, all completed the post-assessments and returned for the final interview. Each was interviewed individually.

The parents' response was shocking. It is not a word I use lightly after 30 years in the field and literally thousands of parent meetings. The glowing remarks and showering of praise from exuberant parents were unsettling. One after another, parents detailed the changes in their children. The most striking declaration came from the mother of the child with Tourette syndrome, "Matthew stopped having tics." She described how she even reduced his medication to "next to nothing." It was Christmas, and they had "the best holiday ever." She made a point to inform me that normally children's tics worsen during the holidays. She pleaded for the program to continue.

Another intriguing report came from the mother of the fourth grade boy who remarked about not feeling crazy. She informed me that her son had a severe case of irritable bowel syndrome (IBS). The child soiled his clothes and had to be taken home daily to bathe and redress before returning to school. While in the program, the accidents stopped. Another boy bit his fingernails until they bled; during the program, he had nails.

Near the close of the interviews, a parent reported without prompting that her son had started cleaning his bedroom. I interrupted the mother to suggest that whatever triggered that change likely had nothing to do with the program. Shortly thereafter, the last parent entered the room. When asked if she had observed any changes, she gleefully announced that her son had begun cleaning his bedroom. I inquired and she declared that she had not discussed the matter with any of the other parents.

Undeniably, the children were capable of participating and the outcomes were positive. My enthusiasm was revived. Despite the parents' pleas and my formal request, the program, however, was discontinued. I left the school system and redirected my time and energy. I committed to identifying the common denominator that could stop tics, control bowels, and encourage a child to clean his room.

There were several steps on the pathway to discovery. At the onset of the pursuit, I shared my findings with a respected colleague, a veteran special education director. Without hesitation and in a jocular, sarcastic tone, he responded, "Poppycock! Snake oil." In spite of his skepticism, I knew I was onto something extraordinary. I had been around the block too many times to not recognize what ordinarily happens. It actually was far more a question of why, not if, that perplexed me.

There was a dearth of research devoted to stress in children in general and even less on stress in children with autism. I had to rely heavily on reasoning and employed problem-solving strategies. Documentation existed indicating that meditation reduces stress, and tai chi is recognized as a meditative practice. I knew all of the improvements occurred after introducing the meditative exercises. I was not aware, however, of any documentation linking stress and the symptoms of autism or Tourette syndrome. The nail biting and IBS could stem from anxiety which would link them to stress, but this did not link them to children with special needs. Furthermore, I could not account for the diminishing tics, the "not feeling crazy" comment, nor the cleaner bedrooms. I needed more information to connect the dots.

I began exploring and found research conducted on the topic of stress in children with autism. In her pioneering work, Dr. Blythe Corbett at UC Davis determined there was an atypical response to stressors in children with autism (Corbett et al., 2006). Hopeful, I searched for "stress in children with Tourette syndrome" to account for the decrease in tics, but found nothing. Meanwhile, I had apparently sparked the curiosity of my skeptical colleague who called to tell me he had met an assistant school superintendent who had Tourette syndrome. My colleague shared my findings with him and then asked if he could pass on my contact information. Shortly after I had agreed, the gentleman called. I found him difficult to understand due to his frequent vocal tics. Over the course of our discussion, however, it became clear that he was upset with my claims. He informed me that he was actively involved in the Tourette syndrome community nationally and locally and he had "never heard of such a thing" as tai chi reducing tics. But nonetheless, he acknowledged that when concentrating on something, like shooting foul shots, his tics would temporarily stop. He remarked about a surgeon with Tourette syndrome who stops having tics while operating on patients. This information indicated there were psychological components associated with tics. Once he learned, however, that the boy in the study had remained on medication (regardless of the drastically reduced dosage and the fact that the medication was not controlling his tics prior to the intervention), he immediately dismissed my findings and somehow attributed them to the medication. A few months had passed since I had become aware of Dr. Corbett's work. Distressed from the call, I reentered "Tourette syndrome, stress, children" in the Google Scholar search bar. To my delight she had just published another article; this time she found an abnormal stress response in children with Tourette syndrome (Corbett et al., 2008) I forged ahead. I felt compelled to share my findings with others who might offer insights. Dr. David Amaral, President of the International Society for Autism Research and a colleague of Blythe Corbett's, was speaking at the nearby Children's Hospital of Philadelphia (CHOP). Prior to his conference in Philadelphia, I contacted him. He generously agreed to meet with me to discuss my work. At the time, genetics was the hottest topic in the search for the cause of autism. Current research focuses on a combination of genetic and environmental factors. During our discussion, I shared the results of my work and suggested perhaps the meditative exercises altered the children's genes. With a roll of the eyes, he quickly retorted that "almost anything can alter genes." As he was departing, I handed him a research article that detailed the number and specific genes that were altered after employing a stress reduction intervention. After a quick glance at the paper, Dr. Amaral turned on his heels and remarked, "Maybe you are onto something." The meeting with Amaral was a boost; after all, "maybe" was a step-up from "poppycock" and "snake oil".

My work was intended to be a feasibility study conducted to explore the practicality of implementing a meditative exercise with children who have special needs. The study had relatively few participants and no control group-both obvious limitations but less important in a feasibility study. Regardless, the study yielded noteworthy, remarkable outcomes from standardized instruments pre- and post-intervention. I had conducted psychometric evaluations for years and never found this remarkable of a response-to -intervention (RTI). In my ongoing discussions further objections were raised. It was justifiably argued that the study had not been replicated and that I had been the only trainer to execute the intervention. To remedy these issues, I moved forward to replicate the study and use different trainers.

The second study extended the population to include younger children and girls. Knowing that early intervention often yields more fruitful results, I included children as young as six years old. I recruited a group of four professionals with diverse backgrounds in education to conduct the program. I trained the program leaders using the original protocol that I had developed. Minor modifications had been made to a few exercises in the program, but the format was essentially the same. In the introductory seminar for the second study, parents were invited to meet the new trainers and were given an overview of the program. Of the 22 parents attending the seminar, 21 returned with their children for training. As in the initial study, the children's attendance remained over 90%. A number of parents commented that they would not leave for weekend outings until their child had completed the Saturday morning sessions. As in the original study, the new trainers worked in pairs with one leading the exercises and the other guiding and encouraging the children. A school counselor had assisted me during the original program. The results of the second study were similar to the first. The children were able to participate and there were significant improvements across several categories. I added an anxiety measure to the battery of assessments in the second study. Outcomes indicated anxiety was particularly responsive to treatment. Parents claimed their children were "more focused, less impulsive" and more willing to take direction. Further evidence emerged that social skills were also impacted. The children, who were strangers prior to the program, without my awareness were having "play dates" in each other's homes. On an initial interview one mother remarked that her son had no friends. She teared up while sharing with me that he had no friends to invite for a birthday party. She told me later in the program, and after the fact, that the tai chi group had gathered at this boy's home for a pool party to celebrate his birthday. Additionally, the participants, independent of adult direction, created and structured a game they played routinely at the end of the sessions; they often needed parents' coaxing to leave.

The second study confirmed that the program could be replicated and include younger children. It also demonstrated that the training could be conducted by other professionals. Consistent with the first study, there was a range of remarkable outcomes. There was magic, but it was not my magic. Data from both feasibility studies are detailed in Chapter 19.

Even with the replication of studies, there was no apparent rhyme nor reason for the improvements. I was flabbergasted and with little else to go on, I shifted my focus to acquiring a better understanding of the concept of stress. I needed to determine if stress reduction might truly offer a viable explanation for the changes in the children. New research emerged that began providing answers. Stress is far more complex than previously understood. Dr. Bruce McEwen, an internationally renowned expert on stress, was a neuroendocrinologist at the Rockefeller Institute. Prior to his recent death, he authored over 800 articles on stress and the brain. After one of his conferences I approached him regarding my work. He expressed an interest and graciously offered to mentor me. His influence is evident throughout this book. His classic book, "The End of Stress as We Know It," provides a broad overview with an emphasis on the physiology of stress. His former student and also a brilliant scholar, Dr. Robert Sapolsky, is a neuroendocrinologist at Stanford. Sapolsky also details the physiology of stress in his book, "Why Zebras Don't Get Ulcers." He narrates a compelling documentary produced by National Geographic that I would highly recommend, "Stress -Portrait of a Killer." These resources provided me with a clearer conceptualization that the deleterious consequences of stress are much greater than previously understood. It was generally accepted that stress was bad for you, but evidence that stress hormones altered brain structure and genes was revolutionary. These structural changes were capable of causing and exacerbating a range of symptoms and negatively impacting behavior. The most frequently used biomarker for stress is the glucocorticoid, cortisol. Glucocorticoids produce an array of effects in response to stress. Because excessive stress can cause a realm of serious problems (even life-threatening ones), it logically followed that allaying stress might alleviate them. Eureka! Relieving stress could potentially improve symptoms of autism and other disabilities.

Central to understanding how this could possibly occur involved examining three brain regions primarily responsible for the stress response. The negative impact of stress on these brain regions was being documented by research using magnetic resonance imaging (MRI). Structural alterations in these brain regions could impact a range of symptoms and behaviors many of which mimicked the defining characteristics of autism. Details can be found in Chapter 8.

My earlier speculations connecting stress and symptoms of children with disabilities needed to be validated or discarded. I committed to an in-depth exploration of research related to stress. After a decade of investigation, assisted by the research efforts of neuroscientists, medical personnel, and psychologists, answers emerged. Findings from over a thousand peer-reviewed studies unscrambled matters, piece by piece. The highlights served as the framework for this book. Some findings provided giant leaps forward, others filled in gaps. The unreasonable became logical. The unexpected became predictable. Among those findings it has been determined that stress in the general population differs from the stress of those with autism. It is important to note that the stress response of those with autism is more likely to malfunction. The consequences are substantive and these differences need to be distinguished for diagnostic and treatment purposes. Many of the concepts in this book apply to a range of ages and disabilities including ADHD, Tourette syndrome and anxiety disorders. The findings that follow, however, more specifically focus on the stress of children with autism.

Historically, we have treated symptoms of autism and the consequences of stress independently, unaware of the complex interrelationship between the two. The stress response in those with autism malfunctions beginning at birth and continues to do so throughout life. Stress and autism are tightly interwoven. This revelation dictates a paradigm shift in treatment and prevention. An overview of evidence-based research for treatment is presented in the last section of this book. First, however, acquiring a better understanding of the complexities of stress can assist in appreciating the overwhelming stress of those with autism.

Chapter 2
DEFINING STRESS

Defining stress is like juggling Jell-O. I find that most people, when asked to define stress, reply with the causes of their stress or how badly stress makes them feel. The concept of stress is elusive and difficult to grasp, but there are key elements that define it. Dr. McEwen's definition appears to capture the essence of stress:

"Stress may be defined as a threat, real or implied, to the psychological or physiological integrity of an individual" (McEwen, 1999).

Stress threatens our well-being. It is a negative force with the potential to harm us. If it is not negative, then it is not stress. A key component in defining stress is threat. Stress occurs when we are threatened either physically or psychologically. If someone were to hold a knife to our throat or we were given a mathematics test to perform in front of others, both likely would create stress. Our ability to cope with stressors can yield positive or negative outcomes. Our reactions to stressors depend upon a number of factors including our available resources and training. One can be trained to more effectively cope with stress. More effective methods of addressing stress are detailed later.

McEwen states that stress can be real or implied. I was skeptical. Can stress that isn't real actually be stressful? I became convinced when one day I was sitting quietly and found myself recalling a traumatic event. I noticed my heart racing and my stomach flipping. I acknowledged that I can also experience similar reactions when anticipating future events. While waiting in the reception room for a doctor's appointment, I will find myself growing anxious. Stress can occur in the present, be recalled from the past, and surface when dreading a future event.

The final portion of the definition indicates stress can be threatening either psychologically or physically. Generally speaking, my perceptions are that we associate stress with psychological events. Stress, however, can be generated when physical conditions are extreme including lights that are too bright and noises that are too loud. Physical stressors that trigger sensory reactions are particularly potent for those with autism.

Sapolsky has advanced that humans, uniquely, can get stuck in a state of chronic stress (Sapolsky, 2004). It is widely recognized that stress causes and exacerbates physical and psychological problems in the general population. According to a survey conducted in 2017 by the American Psychological Association (APA, 2017), a sizable proportion (approximately 20 percent) of Americans report experiencing extreme stress; three in ten Americans say their stress has increased in the past year. Stress is out of control.

Children with autism are plagued by stress. It impacts all aspects of their life, and if you don't believe me, ask their mothers. Evidence presented throughout this book substantiates that stress in those with autism is more frequent, intense, and enduring than in typical children. There is, however, no mention of stress under the category of autism in the Diagnostic and Statistical Manual of Mental Disorders, Fifth Edition (DSM-V). This manual is published by the American Psychiatric Association and provides the standard criteria for classifying disabilities. The DSM also fails to mention anxiety in those with autism, even though abnormally high anxiety rates impact an estimated 40% of this population (van Steensel et al., 2011). Stress is not anxiety, but stress causes anxiety and stress can cause so much more (Mitra et al., 2008). Stress can wreak havoc on thinking, sleeping, digesting, and interacting. It does so in those with autism. Defining symptoms of this disorder and co-morbid conditions associated with autism can be caused and exacerbated by stress. Fortunately, issues with the DSM diagnostic criteria are being addressed by the National Institute of Mental Health (NIMH). The NIMH has launched a project referred to as the Research Domain Criteria (RDoC) Initiative with the mission to transform diagnosis. NIMH is recommending genetics, imaging, and cognitive science be incorporated in the diagnosis. The goal of the RDoC Initiative is to lay the foundation for a new classification system that is more biologically based, one with a research framework that does not rely on disorder-based categories. The evidence in this book meets the new criteria. Autism needs to be redefined and stress needs to be a part of the new diagnostic criteria.

Chapter 3
THE MALFUNCTIONING STRESS RESPONSE OF AUTISM

An appropriate stress response is a healthy and necessary part of life; it is a powerful and sophisticated defense mechanism that mobilizes the body to cope with threatening situations. As part of that response, energy is shunted to body parts that need it most, memory is enhanced, and immune functions improve, but only in the short term. This dynamic regulatory process adapts to the demands of stress, and the body returns to normal once the challenge of the stressors is met, a process known as allostasis. When this protective response malfunctions or becomes overloaded by an abundance of stressors, "allostatic load" occurs. This overload can initiate a proliferation of interactive and detrimental consequences to the brain that among other outcomes can compromise future stress resiliency (McEwen & Gainers, 2010; McEwen & Lasley, 2002). Allostatic load characterizes the state of stress in those with autism.

The brain is the key organ primarily responsible for reacting to and recovering from stress. The stress response is orchestrated by a large network of interactive neural structures in the central, peripheral, and endocrine systems (Chuck et al., 2013; McEwen & Lasley, 2002, O'Connor et al., 2000). Normally, an effective stress response is a short-term operation (de Kloet et al., 2005). Essentially, the stress response occurs in three separate and distinct stages.

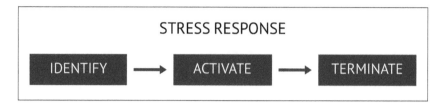

- Stage I Identify - The brain identifies the threat.
- Stage II Activate - A physiological response to the stressor occurs. This is commonly referred to as the "fight or flight" stage.
- Stage III Terminate - The body effectively addresses the stressor and the stress response ends. All systems return to normal.

It has been determined that the cortisol signaling system as part of the human stress response is far more complex and nuanced than originally thought. In order to effectively treat stress and prevent its detrimental effects, it is important to recognize the role of the stress response. A clearer picture emerges when the stress response is viewed in its entirety. An overview of the healthy, properly functioning stress response follows along with a comparison of the abnormal, malfunctioning stress response in children with autism. Malfunctions can occur during any stage and appear to occur in each stage of the stress response in those with autism. The overload of stressors and the malfunctioning stress response create the perfect storm. "It is neither normal nor inevitable for a system designed to protect us to become a threat in and of itself" (McEwen & Lesley, 2002), but this is exactly what is occurring in children with autism.

Chapter 4
STAGE I - IDENTIFY

Stressors in those with autism occur more often, are more intense, and last longer. Stressors evoke the stress response. Frequency, intensity, and duration are factors that impact the potency of a stressor. Children with autism characteristically perceive stimuli differently than their typically developing (TD) peers (Hirstein et al., 2001). Stimuli that likely elicit a stress response in children with autism including toddlers often elicit no reaction in a typical child. Conversely, there are also times when a typical child will react to something that goes virtually unnoticed in a child with autism. At a very young age, children with autism have stressors that differ from typical children. A variety of stimuli that typically elicit fearful and threatening reactions in toddlers did not elicit reactions in toddlers with autism. A toy dinosaur making a loud noise, a plastic moving spider, and a strange man dressed in a mask who stood in close proximity to the toddlers all elicited the stress response in typical children. The toddlers with autism were unresponsive (Macari et al., 2018). To the contrary, routine social interactions for children with autism are consistently shown to be more stressful for them than their typical peers, beginning at an early age. Toddlers with autism show significantly more severe signs of anxiety and avoidance of others in social interactions than controls (Davis III et al., 2010). Children with autism are reluctant to initiate play and are much more likely to reject invitations to play from others. Those who are less socially competent and have fewer friendships are at greater risk of being victimized. An estimated 75% of the children with autism are victims of bullies, a rate four times higher than that of their nondisabled peers. The threats of bullies are stressful. As those with autism become older, they engage in even less social interaction, and social stressors appear to be even more threatening (Corbett et al., 2010; Little, 2001; Schupp et al., 2013).

Reactions to social stressors by children with autism also differ from their typical peers in structured settings. When performing in front of others, it is normal to experience what has been termed "social evaluative threat." This threat is normally the most likely psychological stressor to activate the release of stress hormones (Dickerson & Kemeny, 2004). The stakes are high. Individuals are judged on their ability to perform. The level of our accomplishments influences our social status-recall the popularity of the star football player from high school. Children low in social competence are particularly likely to react to social evaluative threat (Schmidt, 1999). Reactions in those with autism would, therefore, be expected. Their reactions to social pressures, however, are unpredictable. Sometimes they react, sometimes they don't (Taylor & Corbett, 2014). Social evaluative threat in adolescents with autism did not elicit a significant change in cortisol as occurred in typically developing adolescents (Edmiston et al., 2017). I recall observing a child with autism in a regular classroom setting. While at his desk the ten-year-old boy pulled out an egg salad sandwich from his lunch bag around 10:00 AM. While he unwrapped the sandwich on his desk, the crinkling noise and distinctive odor of eggs drew the attention of his classmates. The boy nonchalantly sat and ate the entire sandwich without batting an eye.

Reactions to sensory stimuli also differ markedly from normal in those with autism. It was noted earlier that their reactions are extreme. As many as 95% of those with autism have sensory issues ranging from hyperreactivity to hyporeactivity, particularly to auditory, visual, and tactile stimuli (Ben-Sasson et al., 2008; Lane et al., 2012). Sensory overload can be detected by observing the actions of the child who may cup their ears to deaden sound, shade their eyes from overhead lights, and cry in anguish from the irritation of a clothing tag. These reactions can be occurring while other children in close proximity show no signs of distress (Matsushima et al., 2016; Schaaf et al., 2015).

Affectionate touch is normally soothing and modulates stress. Adults with autism exhibit disruptions in the neural mechanisms for processing affectionate touch and the more severe the autism, the more diminished the response (Voos et al., 2013). Beginning in infancy reactions to sensory stimuli appear to be different from normal in those who will later be diagnosed with autism. Parents of typically developing infants appear to receive positive feedback from the infant that encourages them to continue their gentle stroking for the first two years. In contrast, the parents of infants who later are diagnosed with autism discontinue stroking and switch from affectionate touch to stimulating activities like tickling, making faces, or shaking rattles between six and twelve months after birth (Apicella et al., 2013). Sensations that are easily tolerated by others can be stressful for those with autism (Stiegler & Davis, 2010). One can safely conclude their reactions are unpredictable and differ from typically developing children.

Chapter 5
STAGE II - ACTIVATE

Not only can children with autism have more abundant and salient stressors, but evidence indicates their ability to address stress is compromised. The autonomic nervous system (ANS) and, when necessary, the hypothalamic-pituitary-adrenal (HPA) axis jointly address stressors (Ulrich-Lai & Herman, 2009). Both systems malfunction in children with autism. This type of malfunctioning can be identified at birth (Nagarajan et al., 2016; Sah,et al., 2003). In a normal, healthy response to stress, a series of predictable biological events occurs to address a threat. The ANS and HPA axis stress circuits appear to react independently in response to the specific demand and seriousness of the stressor.

Autonomic Nervous System (ANS). The stress response begins when the brain perceives a stressor. The ANS provides the most immediate response to a stressor by initiating rapid alterations in physiological states. If the stressor is life-threatening, like heavy blood loss or lack of oxygen, this immediately activates a reflexive response to the stressor. The ANS releases the hormones epinephrine (adrenalin) and norepinephrine (noradrenalin). The body prepares for vigorous and sudden action, a phenomenon widely recognized as the "fight or flight" response. The ANS initiates and terminates the stress response through its sympathetic and parasympathetic branches. When operating properly, the sympathetic and parasympathetic systems balance one another, first by adapting to the demands of stressors, then relaxing and returning the system to normal. Reactions of the ANS in children with autism often range between two unhealthy extremes of hyperarousal or hypoarousal.

Hyperarousal. Highly elevated autonomic arousal can be caused by a sustained and exaggerated sympathetic reaction or conversely an insufficient or absent parasympathetic response (Ming et. al. 2005). The sympathetic system initiates profound changes often associated with stress including elevated heart rates, excessive perspiration, and gastrointestinal disorders (Goodwin et al., 2006). Evidence of autonomic arousal was found in children with autism (Daluwatte et al., 2013; Hirstein et al., 2001). Resting heart rates of children with autism were 96 bpm compared to 74 bpm in typical controls (Goodwin et al., 2006). Interrupting an activity of a child with autism can create bursts of extremely large, hyperresponsive sympathetic surges followed by agitation (Hirstein et al., 2001). Chronic hyperarousal sustains "fight or flight" behaviors (Kushki et al., 2013; Hirstein et al., 2001).

Hypoarousal. Abnormally low arousal of the ANS can also occur. While resting, lower electrodermal activity (EDA), a measurement of sympathetic arousal, was detected in children with autism compared to typical controls (Panju et al., 2015; Bujnakova et al., 2016). Children with autism who had low EDA and high anxiety had significantly more severe symptoms than those in the low-anxiety group and the controls (Panju et al., 2015). Those with autism and hyporesponsivity were found to more frequently engage in self-injurious behavior (Hirstein et al., 2001).

Hypothalamic-Pituitary-Adrenal Axis (HPA). The HPA axis is the second major stress regulation system (Sapolsky et al., 2000). Operations of the HPA axis begin with the brain triggering a cascade of hormones in reaction to a stressor. The hypothalamus releases the main driver of the stress hormone system, corticotropin releasing hormone (CRH), into the bloodstream. This hormone binds to receptors in the pituitary gland. The pituitary is activated and then secretes a different hormone, adrenocorticotropin hormone (ACTH), which binds with receptors in the adrenal gland. The adrenal gland then re-leases cortisol. Cortisol is the end-product of the HPA axis activity. Cortisol levels have a direct influence on brain circuits including emotion regulation. Cortisol levels can be detected in saliva and normally follow a clear, pre-dictable circadian rhythm with levels that are highest in the morning and decline throughout the day (Vaillancourt et al., 2008). Irregular rhythms are documented in children and adolescents with ASD (Brosnan et al., 2009; Corbett et al., 2009).

Excessive stress or a malfunctioning of the HPA axis can trigger the release of excessively high amounts of cortisol (hypercortisolaemia), or insufficiently low quantities (hypocortisolaemia). Either can wreak havoc, and both ex-tremes frequently are detected in children with autism (Barrington, 2001; Davis et al., 2006; Karemaker et al., 2008; Corbett et al., 2009). Abnormal amounts of cortisol can alter brain neuroarchitecture and cause changes in the cell nucleus that regulates gene expression (Fuchs & Czéh, 2006; Lu-cassen et al., 2014; McEwen & Lasley, 2002).

Both the ANS and HPA axis address the stressors in our daily lives. The over-load of stressors generated from sensory impairments and social interactions in those with autism chronically activates these systems. Moreover, both sys-tems fail to effectively address the overabundance of stressors. A review of fifty-seven studies that assessed the physiological reactivity of the ANS and HPA axis to sensory and social stressors in those with autism found abnormal reactivity (higher or lower than normal) in over 65% of the studies (Lydon et al., 2014). Highlights follow.

Sensory Stimuli. Both the sympathetic and parasympathetic branches of the ANS are ineffective in modulating reactions to sensory stimuli in children with autism (Schaaf et al., 2013; Woodward et al., 2012). This is a central issue and reflected in the prevalence of sensory problems in children with autism, which has been estimated to be as high as 95% (Lane et al., 2012). Extreme reactions to sensory stimuli, referred to as sensory over-responsivity

(SOR), range from hyperactive to hyporeactive (Ben-Sasson et al., 2008; Lane et al., 2012; LeDoux, 2003). Manifestations of SOR may include avoiding or highly reacting to visual stimuli, noises, and touching (Green et al., 2013; Schaaf et al., 2015).

Social Interactions. During social interactions, the ANS reacts differently in children with autism as compared to their typical peers. Normally the ANS does not react while children interact with familiar persons, but with autism there is sympathetic arousal even while interacting with familiar persons (Neuhaus et al., 2015). Skin conductance response (SCR) is a measure of physiological arousal that increases with activities involving emotional processing (Patterson II et al., 2002). The SCR was determined to be significantly higher in those with autism than for TD peers under a variety of social conditions (O'Haire et al., 2015). Routine social interactions for children with autism are more stressful than for their TD peers beginning at an early age and increasing as they grow older (Corbett et al., 2010; Schupp et al., 2013; Taylor & Corbett, 2014). Ineffective parasympathetic activation is also evident during their social interactions. In children with autism, lower than normal parasympathetic activity (which is important in relaxation) has been associated with difficulties in recognizing emotional cues of others and a greater reluctance to interact with unfamiliar people as compared to controls (Bal et al., 2010; Van Hecke et al., 2009).

The HPA axis also reacts to the stress of social interactions. Children with autism were observed to engage in fewer social overtures and spend less time interacting than their TD peers during play. While interacting with peers, those with autism had significantly higher levels of cortisol than their TD peers (Corbett et al., 2010). Lower-functioning children with autism had higher cortisol levels that were significantly associated with more severe impairments in social interactions (Tordjman et al., 2014).

To summarize, the first two stages of the stress response, initiation and activation, malfunction in those with autism. Not only are children with autism bombarded by an inordinate number of stressors, but their systems do not effectively address them, adding insult to injury. Their systems become over-taxed and need to shut down. This final stage, when the stress response desperately needs to terminate, also malfunctions.

Chapter 6
STAGE III - TERMINATE

Typically, once a threat has passed, the stress response ends and the body returns to normal. Ending the stress response is essential in avoiding the harm caused by prolonged stress. Normally, mechanisms that control over-responding are activated to avoid excessive stress hormones from being released (Czéh et al., 2008; Pascucci et al., 2007). The stress response, however, is not being effectively curtailed in those with autism. This places these individuals at greater risk for a host of physical and psychological problems including symptoms associated specifically with this disorder. Termination of the stress response, like activation, is highly complex. The two major systems that normally regulate stress are the ANS and HPA axis, and each shuts down the stress response differently.

The arousal of the ANS caused by a stressor is offset by the parasympathetic system. The parasympathetic system triggers the relaxation response which is the protective physiological counteraction to the stress response. The relaxation response decreases heart rate, lowers blood pressure, and alters EEG patterns. Normally, it promotes a state of calmness and attenuates the sympathetic system (Bal et al., 2010; Esch et al., 2003; Lazar et al., 2000; Manzoni et al., 2008; Ming et al., 2005). Not only do children with autism generally appear to experience hyperarousal of the sympathetic nervous system, but evidence indicates their parasympathetic system does not function properly either. Lower-than-normal parasympathetic activity that interferes with the relaxation process occurs in those with autism (Bal et al., 2010; Ming et al., 2005; Daluwatte et al., 2013).

The release of cortisol generated by the HPA axis also needs to be regulated. Ordinarily, cortisol secretion has a diurnal rhythm that peaks in the morning and diminishes throughout the day (Jacobson & Sapolsky 1991). The diurnal rhythm of those with autism is abnormal with cortisol levels remaining significantly higher throughout the evening hours (Muscatel & Corbett 2017). The regulatory systems that normally terminate stressors malfunction in those with autism.

There are three brain regions that are instrumental in the regulation of the stress response. A detailed review of their roles regarding stress in autism follows.

Chapter 7
THREE BRAIN REGIONS

The brain initiates and terminates the stress response. The three brain regions primarily responsible for stress regulation are the amygdala, hippocampus, and prefrontal cortex (PFC). The effectiveness of these regions in detecting and reacting to threats may dictate whether or not we survive.

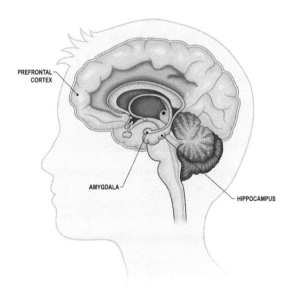

Our senses alert us to things that are potentially dangerous- too hot, too close, too bright, or too mean. We immediately react to life-threatening stressors. Our brains provide us with the ability to sense, reason, and recall when coping with stressors. The neural circuitry of the three main regions that address stress, however, is particularly vulnerable to harm caused by excessive stress hormones. If the stress response is chronically activated by unremitting stressors, then a proliferation of interactive and detrimental consequences to brain structure and functioning can occur (McEwen & Gianaros, 2010; McEwen & Lasley, 2002). Stress can quickly and severely damage the brain (McEwen & Lasley, 2002). The neuroarchitecture of the brain can be altered by excessively high or insufficiently low levels of stress hormones. Extremes in cortisol secretion can have deleterious effects on neurons, particularly those in the hippocampus, amygdala, and prefrontal cortex. Each of these regions is structurally altered and malfunctions in those with autism. The degree of structural alterations is positively correlated with the severity of their symptoms (Juranek et al., 2006; Schumann et al., 2009).

With autism, head circumference at birth is below normal, but suddenly between 1 to 2 months and again at 6 to 14 months, it enlarges rapidly. Ninety percent of children with autism between 2 and 3 years old were found to have brain volumes larger than normal (Courchesne et al., 2003). This overgrowth effects specific regions of the brain. The lobes with overgrowth contain the three brain regions critical in the stress response. MRI research on autistic 2 to 4-year-olds shows the frontal and temporal lobes, particularly the amygdala, as sites of peak overgrowth. This time frame is the most important period in human life for the formation of the neural wiring patterns that make development of higher-order social, emotional, and communicative functions possible (Courchesne et al., 2007).

The neuroarchitecture of the brain can be altered by excessively high or insufficiently low levels of cortisol (Fuchs et al., 2006; Lucassen et al., 2014; McEwen & Lasley, 2002). Structural changes to brain neuroarchitecture include changes in neuron length. Extremes in cortisol levels can cause an overgrowth or retraction of neurons altering brain volume and interfering with subsequent brain network processing. Dendritic length, number of branches, and spine density may increase or decrease; dendritic hypertrophy occurs with significant increases and dendritic hypotrophy/neuronal atrophy with substantial decreases. Alterations in brain neuroarchitecture can disrupt neuronal connections and influence subsequent brain network processing (Fuchs et al., 2006; McEwen & Gianaros, 2010; Mitra & Sapolsky, 2008; Vyas et al., 2002; Zohar et al., 2011). Below: A Normal; B Hypertrophy; C Hypotrophy. Dendritic hypertrophy induced by stress has been observed in real-time. When the soil nematode Caenorhabditis elegans is exposed to stressful conditions, dendritic arborization of its neurons rapidly leads to an exponential increase in total dendritic length and impaired functioning. Stress causes them to grow. When stressful conditions are alleviated, the dendrites retract, and normal functioning is restored (Schroeder et al., 2013). Hypertrophy was observed in rats after being administered just a single dose of corticosterone, the rat-specific glucocorticoid similar to cortisol in humans (Mitra & Sapolsky, 2008). In mice that were genetically bred to display autistic-like behaviors, dendritic overgrowth was found. Excessive branching interferes with neuronal connectivity and the transmitting of information (Cheng et al., 2017).

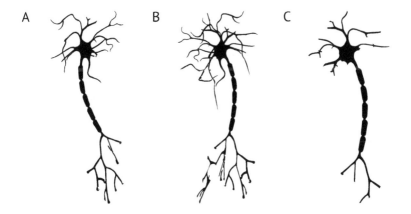

Conversely, dendritic hypotrophy, the decrease or loss of dendrites, has also occurred in mice after a brief exposure to social stress. When mice were exposed to social stress for only one hour on two consecutive days, the length of apical dendrites in the hippocampus was reduced by 77% and the growth of new dendritic branches was slowed (Fuchs et al., 2006). In an earlier study restraint stress of mice over a three-week period caused apical dendrites to atrophy (Watanabe et al., 1992).

Both hypertrophy and atrophy can respectively increase or decrease brain volume and impair functioning (Vyas et al., 2002; Fuchs et al., 2006; Mitra & Sapolsky, 2008; McEwen & Gianaros, 2010; Zohar et al., 2011). Alterations in brain volume, found in the three brain regions that are instrumental in stress regulation, have been documented in children with autism. The functions of these regions and the consequences for those with autism, when the systems do not operate properly, follows.

Prefrontal Cortex. The prefrontal cortex (PFC) represents the pinnacle of evolutionary brain development. Complex, higher-order cognitive abilities, including the executive functions, are generated in this brain region. The executive functions allow us to organize, attend, and exercise self-control. Academic success is largely dependent upon the PFC. Its main function, however, appears to be self-control, think before you act. The PFC interprets social cues and guides us in the avoidance of interpersonal conflict (Mah et al., 2004). Behavioral flexibility, as opposed to rigidity, stems from the PFC. It generates solutions to threatening, stress-evoking situations, e.g., changing hallways when you eye a bully down the corridor.

The PFC is the brain region that is most sensitive to the detrimental effects of stress. The PFC plays an instrumental role in the inhibition of stress, but if the stress is chronic, it responds with structural changes to an even greater degree than other brain regions. These alterations include a reduction in volume and altered or atrophied dendrites. As previously detailed, stress hormones can increase or decrease brain volume. Both acute and chronic stressors produce profound rearrangements of PFC neurons. When functioning properly, the PFC controls and inhibits stress to avoid pathological outcomes (Czéh et al., 2008; Pascucci et al., 2007). The PFC in children with ASD is larger than normal, with an excess of 67% more neurons than TD controls. This "pathological overabundance" of neurons is generated during prenatal life (Courchesne et al., 2011). Structural alterations to the PFC cause a rapid and dramatic loss of prefrontal cognitive abilities. Damage to the PFC produces a profile of distractibility, forgetfulness, impulsivity, poor planning, and hyperactivity (Brennan & Arnsten, 2008). Social inter-actions are also compromised (Brennan & Arnsen, 2008; Mah et al., 2004). Individuals with damaged PFCs display weaknesses in interpersonal judg-ments and problems perceiving social and emotional cues from facial or vocal expressions (Mah et al., 2004). Boys with decreased PFC volume exhibited poor impulse control (Boes et al., 2009). When the PFC malfunctions, inat-tentive, hyperactive and impulsive behaviors emerge.

Hippocampus. The hippocampus is essential in memory formation (McEwen, 1999). It creates memories from your wedding day, stores your zip code, and assists you in finding your car in a parking lot. These are ex-amples of episodic, declarative, and spatial memory, respectively.

In regard to stress, memory is a double-edged sword. Recalling the outcomes of past events can assist in future decision making and prevent repeating prior mistakes that created stress in our lives. But, unfortunately, recalling previous threatening events can also evoke stress, as occurs in post-traumatic stress disorder, (PTSD).

The hippocampus is one of the first regions to be targeted by excessive stress. It is particularly vulnerable to the onslaught of glucocorticoids. Excessive exposures to glucocorticoids during prenatal development and exposure to stress after birth can rapidly damage and kill neurons in the hippocampus (Cai et al., 2008; McEwen, 1999). Damage can occur quickly. Male rats were paired and then separated after only two brief aggressive encounters. The defeated males displayed a 77% reduction in the length of apical den-drites of CA3 hippocampal neurons and had fewer new dendritic branches.

If left in close proximity to the aggressor, deterioration of the victim's brain continued over time (Kole et al., 2004). Victims of bullies have a dysregulation of the HPA axis as indicated by abnormal cortisol levels and higher rates of anxiety (Hansen et al., 2006; Vaillancourt et al., 2008). Bullies selectively target children with autism.

Once damaged by stress hormones, the hippocampus malfunctions. Impairments include misinterpreting and overreacting to future events which further increases stress hormone levels (McEwen 2002).

At the cellular level excessive stress hormones disrupt memory (Conrad, 2010). Normally, the electrochemical activity that occurs between two neurons results in increased synaptic connections which are the foundation of memory. These connections grow stronger with frequent activation. This process of strengthening synapses is known as "long-term potentiation." Stress interferes with the reoccurrence of the signal between neurons (Pavlides et al., 2002). The extent of this disruption depends upon the region of the brain affected. The hippocampus is a region that is particularly vulnerable (Artola et al., 2006, Foy et al., 2011; Pavlides et al., 2002; Shors et al., 1989; Xu et al., 1997). Dendrites retract and spatial memory deficits occur in male rats subjected to chronic restraint stress (McLaughlin et al., 2007).

Not only can stress damage neurons, interfere with memory formation, and cause the stress response to malfunction, it also suppresses the growth of new brain cells. New brain cells are created primarily in the hippocampus through a process known as "neurogenesis" (McEwen, 2006). Prenatal stress in rats induced lifespan reduction of neurogenesis. The normal increase in cell proliferation that occurs, once a new task has been acquired, did not occur in rats who experienced prenatal stress. These rats also had greater difficulty in learning a task that required memory (Lemaire et al., 2000). Postnatal stimulation of the pups, however, counteracts prenatal stress-induced deficits (Lemaire et al., 2006).

The hippocampi of children with autism and children who suffer from PTSD have been found to be abnormal (Carrion et al., 2007). Children with autism, as young as three years old, have hippocampi with increased volumes and altered shapes (Groen et al., 2010; Schumann et al., 2004; Sparks et al., 2002).

Amygdala. Beginning prenatally, the amygdalae of those with autism undergo an abnormal pattern of accelerated growth (Courchesne et al., 2011a). Bilateral amygdalar enlargement has been found in a large sample of 2-year-olds with autism that persisted through 4 years of age (Mosconi et al., 2009). A reversal in this developmental trajectory begins during adolescence. The larger than normal volume is followed by a reduction in size until late middle age (Nacewicz et al., 2006; Schumann & Amaral, 2006; Courchesne et al., 2011). This reversal has been referred to as a "degeneration", suggesting it is not a healthy change (Courchesne et al., 2011). Curiously, this abnormal developmental trajectory also occurs in Tourette Syndrome (TS) (Courchesne et al., 2011; Peterson et al., 2007). Since tics are prevalent in autism as well as TS, the impact of stress on tics will be detailed in Chapter 11.

Stress changes the volume of the basolateral amygdala (BLA) in either direction. An enlargement can be caused by an overgrowth of neurons: dendritic hypertrophy, or a decrease in volume referred to as dendritic hypotrophy or neuronal atrophy (Vyas et al., 2002; Vyas et al., 2003; Mitra et al., 2005). Larger-than-normal amygdala volumes are documented in children whose mothers had higher-than-normal cortisol levels during pregnancy (Buss et al., 2012). Anxiety is associated with decreased amygdala volume in children with autism (Herrington et al., 2017).

The amygdala plays an integral role in both sensory reactions and social interactions. The amygdala is highly responsive to sensory input from all modalities: olfactory, somatosensory, gustatory, visceral, auditory, and visual. It "senses" danger. This brain region alerts us to threats caused by sensory stimuli. In persons with autism, predictably, the amygdala has been found to be more activated. With this subgroup, "habituation", the process by which the system becomes less reactive to a stimuli, is also less likely to occur. They become more stimulated, and it does not diminish or go away as it does with others (Green et al., 2015).

Social interactions also generate activity in the amygdala (Bickart et al., 2014). The amygdala reacts swiftly and efficiently to emotionally charged events, whether real or imagined. It is particularly attuned to threatening social cues, such as an angry face. Within their first week of life, infants normally pay attention to the eyes of other people. When individuals with autism look at the eyes of others, there is a strong hyperactivation of the amygdala, suggesting that for these individuals eye contact generates over-arousal and anxiety (Dalton et al., 2005). Toddlers with autism demonstrate a lack of fixation on the eyes of others; the less the fixation, the greater the social disability (Jones et al., 2008). Children with pediatric generalized anxiety disorder have significantly larger-than-normal amygdala volumes (De-Bellis et al., 2000). These highly anxious children pay more attention to pictures of angry faces; and the more severe their anxiety the greater are their fears of social interactions (Waters et al., 2008). Irritable bowel syndrome presents at rates significantly higher than normal in children with ASD and is directly associated with elevated stress hormones and abnormal amygdala activity (Myers & Greenwood-Van Marveled, 2009).

The three brain regions, the hippocampus, prefrontal cortex (PFC), and amygdala, each play roles in terminating the stress response (Figueiredo et al., 2003; Bhatnagar et al., 2004). The hippocampus normally inhibits excessive cortisol release throughout the day. The PFC normally shuts down the stress response when it has been triggered by psychological stressors (Czéh et al., 2008; Figueiredo et al., 2003; Pascucci et al., 2007). The amygdala typically inhibits responses to novel stressors that no longer pose a threat; it does not terminate reoccurring stressors (Bhatnagar et al., 2004). The regulatory systems that normally terminate stressors fail to operate properly in those with autism.

Chapter 8
HABITUATION

Our bodies come equipped to deal with stressors and our brains determine which need immediate attention. Our systems prioritize those that are life threatening, but the majority of stressors do not pose threat to life or limb. They nevertheless need to be addressed. To avoid overtaxing our systems, we stop reacting to certain stressors.

I vividly recall the first evening in my new home several years ago. A train roared by my bedroom window awakening me from a sound sleep. The blinding light and deafening rumble totally freaked me out. It was indeed stressful. Within a few days the trains continued passing on schedule, but I was sleeping through the night.

We get used to things. As part of adaptation, we have a biological mechanism, known as habituation, that can decrease the neural response to a stimulus when it recurs (Rankin et al., 2008; Turk-Browne et al., 2008). Animals across species habituate; this adaptive process is present early in the life cycle and has been detected as early as the larval stage of zebrafish (Roberts et al., 2012). The ability to habituate is present in humans at birth and continues throughout our lifetimes. Individuals with autism, however, fail to habituate. Stressors can continue to wreak havoc for them long after they have quit being stressful for someone else. There may be no relief. In fact, sensitization may occur, whereby, reactions to essentially the same stressor become even more intense. Reduced habituation is also associated with heightened anxiety (Swartz et al., 2013).

The root of this problem for those with autism may lie in connectivity problems between two brain regions, the prefrontal cortex (PFC) and the amygdala. Stronger connectivity between these two regions predicts greater habituation. Reduced habituation is correlated with greater autism severity (Swartz et al., 2013).

Habituation in autism has been examined in both sensory and social contexts. Sensory overresponsivity (SOR) entails extremely negative reactions to sensory stimuli, and it occurs in the majority of children with autism (Ben-Sasson et al., 2009). Otherwise unnoticed by most children, stimuli such as the clamor in a school cafeteria, tags in clothing, and bright lights can be powerful stressors for children with autism-and they don't get used to them. SOR impacts brain activity in areas responsible for primary sensory processing, emotion regulation, and response to threat. This sensorilimbic activity is most elevated when auditory and visual stimuli are presented simultaneously. This hyperresponsivity is linked to failure to habituate. Habituation is a healthy response to stress. Three groups of youths were administered a mildly aversive stimuli. Two of the groups had autism, the third group did not. Of the youths with autism, one group had SOR. The youths with autism and SOR did not habituate as well as the typical youths. The ability to habituate was also better in the group who had autism, but did not have SOR. Those with autism and SOR had decreased neural habituation to stimuli in sensory cortices and the amygdala compared with the other two groups (Green et al., 2015). Predictability is an important feature of the sensory environment. When stressors are unpredictable, they create greater neuronal activity and habituation is less likely to occur (Herry et al., 2007).

To assess habituation in a social context, pictures of faces with different expressions are presented for viewing. Reactions to faces travel on a subcortical pathway to the amygdala that is a fast lane for rapidly conveying emotional information, particularly threat. Regardless of the facial expression, the amygdalae of children with autism are more highly reactive than controls when viewing faces (Hadjikhani et al., 2017). Not only do they overreact, but they also are less likely to habituate (Kleinhans et al., 2009; Swartz et al., 2013; Tam et al., 2017). Beginning at an early age, toddlers with relatively severe symptoms of autism showed slower habituation to faces than comparison groups. Slower habituation correlated with poorer social skills and verbal ability (Webb et al., 2010). Typical children showed greater connectivity and habituated more readily to facial expressions than children with autism (Swartz et al., 2013). Typical adolescents with higher trait anxiety showed less habituation over repeated exposures than others with less anxiety (Hare et al., 2008). Individuals with autism can appear to be disinterested in others. This may not be the case. Their lack of social interaction may instead stem from finding social stimuli stressful and aversive (Wiggins et al., 2014). Genes influence the degree to which youths with autism react to social stressors as well as their ability to habituate. The serotonin transporter length polymorphic region (5-HTTLPR) polymorphism is an extensively investigated genetic marker of anxiety and personality (Plieger et al., 2014). It impacts those with autism. Three groups of individuals were shown pictures of sad faces. Those with autism were divided into two groups based on their genes. One had a lower-expressing serotonin transporter genotype (5-HTTLPR) than the other group with autism. The third group were TD controls who also had low-expressing serotonin genotypes. The responses of those with autism and those TD controls with low-expressing genotypes were stronger and persisted longer. Results showed those with autism and low expressing genotypes were most responsive to the sad faces and their reactions persisted. Reactions of the amygdala and the failure to habituate were associated with autism and lower expression of 5-HTTLPR (Wiggins et al., 2014). Problems that occur prior to birth can influence the ability to habituate. Male rats are less likely to habituate to HPA activity if they have been exposed to prenatal stress (Bhatnagar et al., 2004).

The potential influence of genes in habituation was also investigated in families, since the presence of autism in one child increases the likelihood that the younger sibling will also have autism. Low-risk infants (those without an older sibling with autism) demonstrated decreased reactions to a noise stressor over time. In contrast, high-risk infants (those who had an older sibling with autism) showed less habituation (Guiraud et al., 2011). Similarly, TD toddlers with older siblings who have autism take longer to habituate than TD toddlers without siblings with autism (Webb et al., 2010).

Not only can stressors for children with autism be more abundant and unrelenting, but the frequent and persistent emotional outbursts that often accompany stressors may cause these children to be misperceived as malingering or overreacting. Since their reactions can be disruptive, they become likely targets for behavioral interventions. Therapies that employ overexposure or desensitization techniques to eliminate reactions to these stressors risk harmful consequences. The behavioral strategies attempt to habituate stressors by repeated presentation of the stressor under altered circumstances, e.g. from a distance, for short time periods, with candy. Regardless of the contrived conditions, the bottom line entails repeatedly presenting the stressor to a child who does not habituate. As detailed earlier, repeated exposure to stressors risks changing the expression of our genes and significantly damaging the structure and functioning of our brains (Perez et al., 2009; Pruessner et al., 2009). More caution addressing stressors in children with autism needs to be exercised.

Chapter 9
ALLOSTATIC OVERLOAD

The stress response promotes adaptation in the short term "allostasis," but the accumulation of unregulated, chronic stress "allostatic load" can become physically and psychologically debilitating, "allostatic overload". This overload predisposes individuals with or without autism to a range of physical and psychological problems that may ultimately be life-threatening. Very late in the writing of this book I came across a model proposed by Dr. McEwen that outlined the factors that contribute to allostatic overload, factors that cause stress to become toxic (McEwen & Gianaros, 2010.) Prior to viewing his outline, I had written on each of the four factors and their relationship with autism. Dr. McEwen had created a model for allostatic overload and my findings regarding the overload of stress in those with autism overlapped without exception.

ALLOSTATIC OVERLOAD - Four major factors (McEwen & Gianaros, 2010)
1. Frequent stressors
2. Failure of HPA axis and ANS to adequately address the stressor
3. Failure to terminate the stress response
4. Failure to habituate to stressors

These factors contribute to toxic stress in those with autism, each ratcheting up stress levels and contributing to their symptoms. Each has been detailed in the opening chapters. In brief:

- *Individuals with autism are bombarded by an inordinate number of stressors.*
- *Both the ANS and HPA axis malfunction in those with autism, and these systems fail to address stressors effectively. Their systems react in extremes.*
- *Their stress response continues to react to stressors. It fails to terminate the stress response and actually may become hyperactive.*
- *Individuals with autism fail to habituate.*

This raises the question of how a system critical to survival could malfunction at so many levels for those with autism with consequences that are monumental.

REFERENCES

CHAPTER 1 - WHAT HAPPENED?

Corbett, B., Mendoza, S., Abdullah, M., Wegelin, J., & Levine, S. (2006). Cortisol circadian rhythms and response to stress in children with autism. Psychoneuroendocrinology, 31(1), 59-68.

Corbett, B., Mendoza, S., Baym, C., Bunge, S., & Levine, S. (2008). Examining cortisol rhythmicity and responsivity to stress in children with Tourette syndrome. Psychoneuroendocrinology. 2008 Jul;33(6):810-20. doi: 10.1016/j.psyneuen. 2008.03.014. Epub 2008 May 19.

Sapolsky, R.M. (2004). Why zebras don't get ulcers (3rd ed.). New York: Holt Paperbacks.

CHAPTER 2 - DEFINING STRESS

American Psychological Association (2017). Stress in America: The State of Our Nation. Stress in AmericaTM Survey.

McEwen, B.S. (1999). Stress and hippocampal plasticity. Annual Review of Neuroscience, 22, 105-122.

Mitra, R., & Sapolsky, R. (2008). Acute corticosterone treatment is sufficient to induce anxiety and amygdaloid dendritic hypertrophy. Proceedings of the National Academy of Sciences, 105(14), 5573-5578.

National Institute of Mental Health. Research Domain Criteria (RDoC).

New York State Psychiatric Institute. DSM-5 and RDoC: Shared Interests. Updated May 14, 2013.

Sapolsky, R.M. (2004). Why zebras don't get ulcers (3rd ed.). New York: Holt Paperbacks.

Van Steensel, F. J. A., Bögels, S. M., & Perrin, S. (2011). Anxiety disorders in children and adolescents with autistic spectrum disorders: A meta-analysis. Clinical Child and Family Psychology Review, 14, 302–317.

CHAPTER 3 - THE MALFUNCTIONING STRESS RESPONSE OF AUTISM

de Kloet, E., Joëls, M., Holsboer, F. (2005). Stress and the brain: from adaptation to disease. Nat Rev Neurosci, 6(6)463-75.

Kushki, A., Drumm, E., Pla Mobarak, M., Tanel, M., Dupuis, A., Chau, T., Anagnostou, E. (2013). Investigating the autonomic nervous system response to anxiety in children with autism spectrum disorders. PLoS ONE, 8(4): e59730; doi:10.1371/journal.pone. 0059730.

McEwen, B.S., & Gianaros, P.J. (2010). Central role of the brain in stress and adaptation: links to socioeconomic status, health, and disease. Annals of the New York Academy of Sciences 1186 (2010) 190-222.

McEwen, B.S., & Lasley, E.N. (2002). The end of stress as we know it. Washington D.C.: John Henry Press.

O'Connor, T.M., O'Halloran, D.J., & Shanahan, F., (2000). The stress response and the hypothalamic-pituitary-adrenal axis: from molecule to melancholia. QJM: An International Journal of Medicine, 93, 323-333

CHAPTER 4 - STAGE I - IDENTIFY

Apicella, R., Chericoni, N., Costanzo, V., Baldini, S., Billeci, L., Cohen, D., & Muratori, F. (2013). Reciprocity in Interaction: A Window on the First Year of Life in Autism. Autism Research and Treatment, doi 10.115/2018/705895.

Ben-Sasson, A., Cermak, S., Orsmond, G., Tager-Flusberg, H., Kadlec, M., & Carter, A. (2008). Sensory clusters of toddlers with autism spectrum disorders: differences in affective symptoms. The Journal of Child Psychology and Psychiatry, 49:817-825.

Corbett, B. A., Schupp, C. W., Simon, D., Ryan, N., & Mendoza, S. (2010). Elevated cortisol during play is associated with age and social engagement in children with ASD. Molecular ASD, 1(1), 13. doi:10.1186/2040-2392-1-13.

Davis III, T., Fodstad, J., Jenkins, W., Hess, J., Moree, B., Dempsey, T., & Watson, J. (2010). Anxiety and avoidance in infants and toddlers with autism spectrum disorders: Evidence for differing symptom severity and presentation. Research in Autism Spectrum Disorders, 4(2), 305-313.

Dickerson S. & Kemeny, M. (2004). Acute stressors and cortisol responses: a theoretical integration and synthesis of laboratory research. Psychol Bulletin 13(3):355-391.

Edmiston, E., Merle, K., & Corbett, B., (2014). Neural and cortisol responses during play with human and computer partners in children with autism. Soc Cogn Affect Neurosci. 10(8): 1074-83. doi: 10.1093/scan/nsu159. Epub 2014 Dec 30.

Hirstein, W., Iversen, P. & Ramachandran, V.S. (2001). Autonomic responses of autistic children to people and objects. Proceedings of the Royal Society B 268, 1883-1888.

Lane, S.J., Reynolds, S., & Dumenci, L. (2012). Sensory overresponsivity and anxiety in typically developing children and children with ASD and ADHD: cause or coexistence? The American Journal of Occupational Therapy, 66, 5, 595-603.

Little, L. (2001). Peer victimization of children with Asperger spectrum disorders. Journal of the American Academy of Child and Adolescent Psychiatry, 40, 995–996.

Macari, S., DiNicola, L., Kane-Grade, F., Prince, E., Vernetti, A., Powell, K. ...& Chawarska, K. (2018). Emotional expressivity in toddlers with autism spectrum disorder. Journal of the American Academy of Child and Adolescent Psychiatry. Vol 57, 11 828-836.

Matsushima, K., Matsubayashi, J., Toichi, M., Funabiki, Y., Kato, T., Awaya, T., & Kato, T. (2016). Unusual sensory features are related to resting-state cardiac vagus nerve activity in ASD. Research in Autism Spectrum Disorders, 2537-46. doi:10.1016/j.rasd.2015.12.006.

Schaaf, R.C., Benavides, T.W., Leiby, B.E., & Sendecki, J.A. (2015). Autonomic dysregulation during sensory stimulation in children with autism spectrum disorder. Journal of Autism and Developmental Disorders, doi 10.1007/s10803-013-1924-6.

Schmidt, L. (1999). Frontal brain electrical activity in shyness and sociability. Psychological Science, 10(4), 316–320. https://doi.org/10.1111/1467-9280.00161

Schupp, C., Simon, D. & Corbett, B. (2013). Cortisol responsivity differences in children with autism spectrum disorders during free and cooperative play. Journal of Autism and Developmental Disorders, 43(10): doi: 10.1007/s10803-013-1790-2.

Stiller, L. & Davis, R. (2010). Understanding sound sensitivity in individuals with autism spectrum disorders. Focus on Autism and Other Developmental Disabilities, 20(10), 1–9.

Taylor, J. and Corbett, B., (2014). A review of rhythm and responsiveness of cortisol in individuals with autism spectrum disorders. Psychoneuroendocrinology, 49, 207-228.

Voos, A. C., Pelphrey, K. A., & Kaiser, M. D. (2013). Autistic traits are associated with diminished neural response to affective touch. Social Cognitive and Affective Neuroscience, 8(4), 378-386. doi:10.1093/scan/nss009.

CHAPTER 5 - STAGE II - ACTIVATE

Bal, E., Harden, E., Lamb, D., Van Hecke, A., Denver, J., & Porges, S. (2010). Emotion regulation in children with autism spectrum disorders: relations to eye gaze and autonomic state. Journal of Autism and Developmental Disorders, 40: 358-370.

Barrington, K. (2001). Meta-analysis: The adverse neuro-developmental effects of postnatal steroids in the preterm infant: a systematic review of RCTs. BMC Pediatrics, 1:1.

Ben-Sasson, A., Ceramic, S., Orsmond, G., Tager-Flusberg, H., Chadic, M., & Carter, A., (2008). Sensory clusters of toddlers with autism spectrum disorders: differences in affective symptoms. The Journal of Child Psychology and Psychiatry, 49:817-825.

Brosnan, M., Turner-Cobb, J., Munro-Naan, Z.,& Jessop, D. (2009). Absence of a normal Cortisol Awakening Response (CAR) in adolescent males with Asperger syndrome (AS). Psychoneuroendocrinology, 34(7), 1095-1100.

Bujnakova, I., Ondrejka, I., Mestanik, M., Visnovcova, Z., Mestanikova, A., Hrtanek, I., ...& Tonhajzerova, I. (2016) Autism spectrum disorder is associated with autonomic underarousal. Physiol Res.,65 (Supplementum 5):S673-S682.PMID: 28006949.

Corbett, B. A., Schupp, C. W., Simon, D., Ryan, N., & Mendoza, S. (2010). Elevated cortisol during play is associated with age and social engagement in children with ASD. Molecular ASD, 1(1), 13. doi:10.1186/2040-2392-1-13.

Corbett, B.A., Schupp, C.W., Levine, S., & Mendoza, S. (2009). Comparing cortisol, stress, and sensory sensitivity in children with autism. Autism Research, 2(1), 39-49.

Daluwatte, C., Miles, J.H., Christ, S.E., Beversdorf, D.Q., Takahashi, T.N., & Yao, G. (2013). Atypical pupillary light reflex and heart rate variability in children with autism spectrum disorder. Journal of Autism and Developmental Disorder, 43:1910-1925.

Davis, E.P., Townsend, E.L., Gunnar, M.R., Guiang, S.F., Lusky, R.C., Cifuentes, R.F., Georgieff, M.K. (2006). Antenatal betamethasone treatment has a persisting influence on infant HPA axis regulation. Journal of Perinatology, 26(3), 147-153.

Fuchs, E., Flugge, G., & Czéh, B. (2006). Remodeling of neuronal networks by stress. Frontiers in Bioscience, 11, 2746-2758.

Goodwin, M., Groden, J., Velicer, W., Lipsitt, L., Baron, M., Hofmann, S.,& Groden, G. (2006). Cardiovascular arousal in individuals with autism. Focus on Autism and Other Developmental Disabilities, 21, 2, 100-123.

Green, S. A., Rudie, J. D., Colich, N. L., Wood, J. J., Shirinyan, D., Hernandez, L., Tottenham, N., Dapretto, M., & Bookheimer, S. Y. (2013). Overreactive brain responses to sensory stimuli in youth with autism spectrum disorders. Journal of the American Academy of Child and Adolescent Psychiatry, 52(11), 1158–1172.

Hirstein, W., Iversen, P. & Ramachandran, V.S. (2001). Autonomic responses of autistic children to people and objects. Proceedings of the Royal Society B 268, 1883-1888.

Karemaker, R., Chevaliers, A., Wolbeek, M., Tersteeg-Kamperman, M., Baerts, W., Veen, S., ... Heijnen, C. (2008). Neonatal dexamethasone treatment for chronic lung disease of prematurity alters the hypothalamus-pituitary-adrenal axis and immune system activity at school age. Pediatrics, 121(4), 870-878.

Kushki, A., Drumm, E., Pla Mobarak, M., Tanel, M., Dupuis, A., Chau, T., & Anagnostou, E. (2013). Investigating the autonomic nervous system response to anxiety in children with autism spectrum disorders. PLoS ONE, 8(4): e59730; doi:10.1371/journal.pone.0059730.

Lane, S.J., Reynolds, S., & Dumenci, L. (2012). Sensory overresponsivity and anxiety in typically developing children and children with ASD and ADHD: cause or coexistence? The American Journal of Occupational Therapy, 66, 5, 595-603.

LeDoux, J., (2003). The emotional brain, fear, and the amygdala. Cellular and Molecular Neurobiology, 23, 727-738.

Lucassen, P., Pruessner, J., Sousa, N., Almeida, O., Van Dam, A., Rajkowska, G., ... & Czeh, B., (2014). Neuropathology of stress. Acta Neuropathology, 127, 109-135.

Lydon, S., Healy, O., Reed, P., Mulhern,T., Hughes, B., & Goodwin, M. (2014). A systematic review of physiological reactivity to stimuli in autism. Developmental Neurorehabilitatio,doi:10.3109/17518423.2014.97175.

McEwen, B.S., & Lasley, E.N. (2002). The end of stress as we know it. Washington D.C.: John Henry Press.

Ming, X., Julu, P.O, Brimacombe, M., Connor, S., & Daniels, M.L. (2005). Reduced cardiac parasympathetic activity in children with autism. Brain & Development, 27:509-516.

Nagarajan, S., Seddighzadeh, B., Baccarelli, A., Wise, L., Williams, M., & Shields, A.(2016). Adverse maternal exposures, methylation of glucocorticoid-related genes and perinatal outcomes: A systematic review. Epigenomics 8(7) DOI: 10.2217/epi.16.9.

Neuhaus, E., Bernier, R., & Beauchaine, T. (2015). Electrodermal response to reward and non-reward among children with ASD. ASD Research: Official Journal of the International Society for ASD Research, 8(4), 357-370. doi:10.1002/aur.1451.

O'Haire, M. McKenzie, S., Beck, A., & Slaughter, V. (2015). Animals may act as social buffers:Skin conductance arousal in children with autism spectrum disorder in a social context. Dev Psychobiol, 57(5):584-95. doi: 10.1002/dev.21310.

Pang, S., Brian, J., Dupuis, A., Anagnostou, E., & Kushki, A. (2015). Atypical sympathetic arousal in children with autism spectrum disorder and its association with anxiety symptomatology. Molecular ASD, 664. doi:10.1186/s13229-015-0057-5.

Panju, S., Brian, J., Dupuis, A., Anagnostou, E., & Kushki, A. (2015). Atypical sympathetic arousal in children with autism spectrum disorder and its association with anxiety symptomatology. Molecular ASD, 664. doi:10.1186/s13229-015-0057-5.

Patterson, J. II, Ungerleider, L. G., & Bandettini, P. A. (2002). Task-independent functional brain activity correlation with skin conductance changes: an fMRI study. Neuroimage, 17(4), 1797-1806.

Sah, P., Faber, E.S.L., Lopez De Armentia, M., & Power, J. (2003). The amygdaloid complex: anatomy and physiology. Physiological Review, 83(3), 803-834.

Sapolsky, R., Romero,,L., & Munck, A. (2000). How do glucocorticoids influence stress responses? Integrating permissive, suppressive, stimulatory, and preparative actions. Endocr Rev.21(1):55-89.

Schaaf, R.C., Benevides, T.W., Leiby, B.E., & Sendecki, J.A. (2015). Autonomic dysregulation during sensory stimulation in children with autism spectrum disorder. Journal of Autism and Developmental Disorders, doi 10.1007/s10803-013-1924-6.

Schupp C., Simon, D. & Corbett, B. (2013). Cortisol responsivity differences in children with autism spectrum disorders during free and cooperative play. Journal of Autism and Developmental Disorders, 43(10): doi: 10.1007/s10803-013-1790-2.

Taylor, J. & Corbett, B., (2014). A review of rhythm and responsiveness of cortisol in individuals with autism spectrum disorders. Psychoneuroendocrinology, 49, 207-228.

Tordjman, S., Anderson, G., Kermarrec, S., Bonnot, O., Geoffray, M., Brailly-Tabard, S., ...Touitou, Y., (2014). Altered circadian patterns of salivary cortisol in low-functioning children and adolescents with autism. Psychoneuroendocrinology 50, 227-245.

Ulrich-Lai, Y. & Herman, J. (2009). Neural regulation of endocrine and autonomic stress responses. Nat Rev Neurosci 10, 397–409 (2009). https://doi.org/10.1038/nrn2647.

Vaillancourt, T., Duke, E., Decatanzaro, D., Macmillan, H., Muir, C., & Schmidt, L.A. (2008). Variation in hypothalamic-pituitary-adrenal axis activity among bullied and non-bullied children. Aggressive Behavior, 34(3), 294-305.

Van Hecke, A.V., Lamb, D., Lebow, J., Bal, E., Harden, E., Kramer, A., ... Porges, S.W., (2009). Electroencephalogram and heart rate regulation to familiar and unfamiliar people in children with autism spectrum disorder. Child Development, 80, 1118-1133.

Woodward, C., Goodwin, M., Zelazo, P., Aube, D., Scrimgeour, M., Ostholthoff, T., & Brickley, M. (2012). A comparison of autonomic, behavioral, and parent-report measures of sensory sensitivity in young children with autism. Research in Autism Spectrum Disorders 6, 1234-1246.

CHAPTER 6 - STAGE III - TERMINATE

Bal, E., Harden, E., Lamb, D., Van Hecke, A.V., Denver, J.W., & Porges, S.W. (2010). Emotion regulation in children with autism spectrum disorders: relations to eye gaze and autonomic state. Journal of Autism and Developmental Disorders, 40: 358-370.

Czéh. B., Perez-Cruz, C., Fuchs, E., & Flügge, G. (2008). Chronic stress-induced cellular changes in the medial prefrontal cortex and their potential clinical implications: Does hemisphere location matter? Behavioural Brain Research, 190(1), 1-13.

Daluwatte, C., Miles, J.H., Christ, S.E., Beversdorf, D.Q., Takahashi, T.N., & Yao, G. (2013). Atypical pupillary light reflex and heart rate variability in children with autism spectrum disorder. Journal of Autism and Developmental Disorder, 43:1910-1925.

Esch, T., Fricchione, G., & Stefano, G. (2003). The therapeutic use of the relaxation response in stress-related diseases. Medical Science Monitor, 9, 23-34.

Jacobson & Sapolsky (1991). The role of the hippocampus in feedback regulation of the hypothalamic-pituitary-adrenocortical axis. Endocr Rev. 1991 May;12(2):118-34.

Lazar, S., Bush, G., Gold, R., Fricchione, G., Khalsa, G., & Benson, H. (2000). Functional brain mapping of the relaxation response and meditation. NeuroReport, 2,7.

Manzoni, G.M., Pagnini, F., Castelnuovo, G., & Molinari, E. (2008). Relaxation training for anxiety: a ten-years systematic review with meta-analysis. BMC Psychiatry, 8(41).

Ming, X., Julu, P.O, Brimacombe, M., Connor, S., & Daniels, M. (2005). Reduced cardiac parasympathetic activity in children with autism. Brain & Development, 27:509-516.

Muscatello, R. & Corbett, B. (2017). Comparing the effects of age, pubertal development, and symptom profile on cortisol rhythm in children and adolescents with autism spectrum. Autism Res. 2018 Jan; 11(1): 110–120. doi: 10.1002/aur.1879.

Pascucci, T., Ventura, R., Latagliata, E.C., Cabib, S., & Puglisi-Allegra, S. (2007). The medial prefrontal cortex determines the accumbens dopamine response to stress through the opposing influences of norepinephrine and dopamine. Cerebral Cortex, 17(12), 2796-2804.

CHAPTER 7 - THREE BRAIN REGIONS

Artola, A., von Frigate, J., Fermont, P., Gispen, W., Schema, L., Kamal, A., & Sprint, B. (2006). Long-lasting modulation of the induction of LTD and LTP in rat hippocampal CA1 by behavioural stress and environmental enrichment. Eur J Neurosci. 2006 Jan;23(1): 261-72.

Bhatnagar, S., Lee, T., & Vining, C., (2004). Prenatal stress differentially affects habituation of corticosterone responses to repeated stress in adult male and female rats. Science Direct. 0018-506X/$.doi:10.106.j-yhbeh.2004.11.019.

Bickart, K., Dickerson, B.,& Barrett, L. (2014). The amygdala as a hub in brain networks that support social life. Neuropsychologia. 2014 Oct; 63: 235–248.

Boes, A.D., Bechara, A., Tranel, D., Anderson, S.W., Richman, L., & Nopoulos, P. (2009). Right ventromedial prefrontal cortex: A neuroanatomical correlate of impulse control in boys. Social Cognitive and Affective Neuroscience, 4(1), 1-9.

Brennan, A.R., & Arnsten, A.F.T. (2008). Neuronal mechanisms underlying attention deficit hyperactivity disorder. Annals of the New York Academy of Sciences, 1129, 236-245.

Buss, C., Davis, E., Shahbaba, B., Pruessner, J., Head, K., and Sandman, C. (2012).

Maternal cortisol over the course of pregnancy and subsequent child amygdala and hippocampus volumes and affective problems. Proc Natl Acad Scie U S A 109: E1312-1319.

Cai, Q., Huang, S., Zhu, Z., Li, H., Li, Q., Jia, N., & Liu, J. (2008). The effects of prenatal stress on expression of p38 MAPK in offspring hippocampus. International Journal of Developmental Neuroscience, 26(6), 535-540.

Carrion, V.G., Weems, C.F., & Reiss, A.L. (2007). Stress predicts brain changes in children: A pilot longitudinal study on youth stress, posttraumatic stress disorder and the hippocampus. Pediatrics, 119(3), 509-516.

Cheng, N., Asshammari, F., Hughes, E., Khanbabaei, M., & Rho, J. (2017). Dendritic overgrowth and elevated ERK signaling during neonatal development in a mouse model of autism. https://doi.org/10.1371/journal.pone.0179409.

Conrad, C. (2010) A critical review of chronic stress effects on spatial learning and memory. Progress in Neuro-Psychopharmaclogy and Biological Psychiatry. Volume 34, Issue 5, 30 June 2010, 742-755.

Courchesne, E., Campbell, K., & Solso, S. (2011). Brain growth across the life span in autism: age-specific changes in anatomical pathology. Brain Research, 1380, 138-145.

Courchesne, E., Carper, R., Akshoormoff, N., (2003). Evidence of brain overgrowth in the first year of life in autism. Journal of the American Medical Association, 290, 337-344.

Courchesne E., Pierce K., Schumann C., Redcay E., Buckwalter, J., Kennedy, D., & Morgan J. 2007). Mapping early brain development in autism. Neuron; 56:399–413.

Czéh. B., Perez-Cruz, C., Fuchs, E., & Flügge, G. (2008). Chronic stress-induced cellular changes in the medial prefrontal cortex and their potential clinical implications: Does hemisphere location matter? Behavioral Brain Research, 190(1), 1-13.

Dalton, K., Nacewicz, B., Johnstone, T., Schaefer, H., Gernsbacher, M., Goldsmith, H. … & Davidson, R.J., (2005). Gaze fixation and the neural circuitry of face processing in autism. Nature Neuroscience, 8, 519-526.

DeBellis, M., Casey, B., Dahl, R., Birmaher, B., Williamson, D., Thomas, K., …& Ryan, N. (2000). A pilot study of amygdala volumes in pediatric generalized anxiety disorder. Biological Psychiatry, 48(1), 51-57.

Figueiredo, H., Bruestle, A., Bodie, B., Dolgas, C., Herman, J., (2003). The medial prefrontal cortex differentially regulates stress-induced c-fos expression in the forebrain depending on type of stressor. European Journal of Neuroscience. 2003;18(8):2357–2364.

Foy, M. (2011). Ovarian hormones, aging and stress on hippocampal synaptic plasticity. Neurobiol Learn Mem. 2011 Feb;95(2):134-44. doi: 10.1016/j.nlm. 2010.11.003.

Fuchs, E., Flugge, G., & Czéh, B. (2006). Remodeling of neuronal networks by stress. Frontiers in Bioscience, 11, 2746-2758.

Green, S., Herandez, L., Tottenham, N., Krasileva, K., Bookheimer, S., & Dapretto, M., (2015). Neurobiology of sensory overresponsivity in youth with autism spectrum disorders. JAMA Psychiatry, 72(8):778-786. Doi:10.1001/jamapsychiatry.2015.0737.

Groen, W., Teluij, M., Buitelaar, J., & Tendolkar, I. (2010). Amygdala and hippocampus enlargement during adolescence in autism. J Am Acad Child Adolesc Psychiatry. 2010 Jun;49(6):552-60. doi: 10.1016/j.jaac.2009.12.023.

Hansen, A.M., Hogh, A., Persson, R., Karlson, B., Garde, A.H., & ⊠rb⊠k, P. (2006). Bullying at work, health outcomes, and physiological stress response. Journal of Psychosomatic Research, 60(1), 63-72.

Herrington, J., Maddox, B., Kerns, C., Rump, K., Worley, J., Bush, J., ...Miller, J. (2017). Amygdala Volume Differences in Autism Spectrum Disorder Are Related to Anxiety. Jour Autism Dev Disord. 2017 Dec;47(12):3682-3691. doi: 10.1007/s10803-017-3206-1.

Jones, W., Carr, K., and Klin, A. (2008). Absence of preferential looking to the eyes of approaching adults predicts level of social disability in 2-year-old toddlers with autism spectrum disorder. Archives of General Psychiatry, 65, 946-954.

Juranek, J., Filipek, P.A., Berenji, G.R., Modahl, C., Osann, K., & Spence, M.A. (2006). Association between amygdala volume and anxiety level: Magnetic resonance imaging (MRI) study in autistic children. Journal of Child Neurology, 21(12), 1051-1058.

Kole, M.H.P., Costoli, T., Koolhaas, J.M., & Fuchs, E. (2004). Bidirectional shift in the cornu ammonis 3 pyramidal dendritic organization following brief stress. Neuroscience, 125(2), 337-347.

Lemaire, V., Koehl, M., Le Moal, M., & Abrous, D.N. (2000). Prenatal stress produces learning deficits associated with an inhibition of neurogenesis in the hippocampus. Proceedings of the American National Academy of Sciences, 97(20), 1132-1137.

Lemaire, V., Lamarque, S., LeMoal, M., Piazza, P., & Abrous (2006) Postnatal stimulation of the pups counteracts prenatal stress-induced deficits in hippocampal neurogenesis. Biological Psychiatry, 59(9), 786-792.

Lucassen, P.J., Pruessner, J., Sousa, N., Almeida, O.F., Van Dam, A.M., Rajkowska, G., ... Czeh, B., (2014). Neuropathology of stress. Acta Neuropathology, 127, 109-135.52.

Mah, L., Arnold, M.C., & Grafman, J. (2004). Impairment of social perception associated with lesions of the prefrontal cortex. American Journal of Psychiatry, 161(7), 1247-1255.

McEwen, B.(1999). Stress and hippocampal plasticity. Annual Review of Neuroscience, 22, 105-122.

McEwen, B., (2006). Plasticity of the Hippocampus: Adaptation to Chronic Stress and Allostatic Load. Annals of the New York Academy of Sciences.

McEwen, B.S., & Gianaros, P.J. (2010). Central role of the brain in stress and adaptation: links to socioeconomic status, health, and disease. Annals of the New York Academy of Sciences 1186 (2010) 190-222.

McEwen, B.S., & Lasley, E.N. (2002). The end of stress as we know it. Washington D.C.: John Henry Press.

McLaughlin, K., Gomez, J., Baran, S., & Conrad, C. (2007). The effects of chronic stress on hippocampal morphology and function: an evaluation of chronic restraint paradigms. Brain Res. 2007 Aug 3;1161:56-64. Pub 2007 Jun 2.

Mitra, R., Jadhav, S., McEwen, B.S., Vyas, A., & Chattarji, S., (2005). Stress duration modulates the spatiotemporal patterns of spine formation in the basolateral amygdala. Proceedings of the National Academy of Sciences of the United States of America, 102, 9371-9376. doi/10.1073/pnas.0504011102.

Mitra, R., & Sapolsky, R. (2008). Acute corticosterone treatment is sufficient to induce anxiety and amygdaloid dendritic hypertrophy. Proceedings of the National Academy of Sciences, 105(14), 5573-5578.

Mosconi, M., Cody-Hazlett, H. Poe, M., Gerig, G., Gimpel-Smith, R., and Piven, J., (2009). Longitudinal study of amygdala volume and joint attention in 2- to 4-year-old children with ASD. Archives of General Psychiatry, 66, 509-516.

Myers, B., & Greenwood-Van Meerveld, B. (2009). Role of anxiety in the pathophysiology of irritable bowel syndrome. Frontiers in Enteric Neuroscience, 3(47), 1-10.

Nacewicz, B., Dalton, K., Johnstone, T., Long, M., McAullff, E.., Oakes, T., ... & Davidson, R., (2006). Amygdala volume and nonverbal social impairment in adolescent and adult males with autism. Archives of General Psychiatry, 63, 1417-1428.

Pascucci, T., Ventura, R., Latagliata, E., Cabib, S., & Puglisi-Allegra, S. (2007). The medial prefrontal cortex determines the accumbens dopamine response to stress through the opposing influences of norepinephrine and dopamine. Cerebral Cortex, 17(12), 2796-2804.

Pavlides, C., Nivon, L., McEwen, B. (2002). Effects of chronic stress on hippocampal long-term potentiation. Hippocampus Volume 12, Issue 2https://doi.org/10.1002/hipo.1116.

Peterson, B.S., Choi, HM. A., Hao, X., Amat, J. A., Zhu, H., Whiteman, R., ... Bansal, R. (2007). Morphologic features of the amygdala and hippocampus in children and adults with Tourette syndrome. Archives of General Psychiatry, 64(11), 1281-1291.

Schroeder, N.E., Androwski, R.J., Rashid, A., Lee, H., Lee, J., and Barr, M.M., (2013). Dauer-specific dendrite arborization in C. elegans is regulated by KPC-1/Furin. Current Biology, 23, 1527-1535.

Schumann, C.M., & Amaral, D.G. (2006). Stereological analysis of amygdale neuron number in autism. The Journal of Neuroscience, 26(29), 7674-7679.

Schumann, C.M., Barnes, C.C., Lord, C., and Courchesne, E., (2009). Amygdala enlargement in toddlers with autism related to severity of social and communication impairments. Biological Psychiatry, 66, 942-949.

Schumann, C.M., Hamstra, J., Goodlin-Jones, B.L., Lotspeich, L.J., Kwon, H., Buonocore, M.H., Amaral, D.G., (2004). The amygdala is enlarged in children but not adolescents with autism; the hippocampus is enlarged at all ages. The Journal of Neuroscience, 24, 6392-6401.

Shors T., Seib T., Levine S., Thompson R. (1989) Inescapable versus escapable stress modulates long-term potentiation in the rat hippocampus. Science 244:224–226.

Sparks, B., Friedman, S., Shaw, D., Aylward, E., Echelard, D., Artru, A. & ...Dager, S. (2002). Brain structural abnormalities in young children with autism spectrum disorder. Neurology. 2002 Jul 23;59(2):184-92.

Vaillancourt, T., Duku, E., Decatanzaro, D., Macmillan, H., Muir, C., & Schmidt, L.A. (2008). Variation in hypothalamic-pituitary-adrenal axis activity among bullied and non-bullied children. Aggressive Behavior, 34(3), 294-305.

Vyas, A., Bernal, S., Chattarji, S., (2003). Effects of chronic stress on dendritic arborization in the central and extended amygdala. Brain Research 965, 290-294.

Vyas, A., Mitra, R., Rao, B.S., & Chattarji, S. (2002). Chronic stress induces contrasting patterns of dendritic remodeling in hippocampal and amygdaloid neurons. The Journal of Neuroscience, 22(15), 6810-6818.

Watanabe, Y., Gould, E. & McEwen, B. (1992). Stress induces atrophy of apical dendrites of hippocampus CA3 pyramidal neurons. Brain Res. 588, 341–345.

Waters, A.M., Mogg, K., Bradley, B.P., & Pine, D.S. (2008). Attentional bias towards angry faces in children with generalized anxiety disorders. Journal of the American Academy of Child and Adolescent Psychiatry, 47(4), 435-442.

Xu L, Anwyl R, Rowan MJ (1997) Behavioural stress facilitates the induction of long-term depression in the hippocampus. Nature 387:497–500.

Zohar, J., Yahalom, H., Kozlovsky, N., Cwikel-Hamzany, S., Matar, M., ... Cohen, H. (2011). High dose hydrocortisone immediately after trauma may alter the trajectory of PTSD: Interplay between clinical and animal studies. Eur. Neuropsychopharmacology Dos: 10.1016/j.euroneuro.2011.06.001.

CHAPTER 8 - HABITUATION

Ben-Sasson, Hen, L., Fluss, R., Cermak, S., Engel-Leger, B., Gal.,E. (2009) A meta-analysis of sensory modulation symptoms in individuals with autism spectrum disorders. J Autism Dev Disord. 2009 Jan;39(1):1-11. doi: 10.1007/s10803-008-0593-3. Epub 2008 May 30.

Bhatnagar, S., Lee, T., & Vining, C., (2004). Prenatal stress differentially affects habituation of corticosterone responses to repeated stress in adult male and female rats. Science Direct. 0018-506X/$.doi:10.106.j-yhbeh.2004.11.019.

Green, S., Herandez, L., Tottenham, N., Krasileva, K., Bookheimer, S., & Dapretto, M., (2015). Neurobioloy of sensory overresponsivity in youth with autism spectrum disorders. JAMA Psychiatry, 72(8):778-786. Doi:10.1001/jamapsychiatry.2015.0737.

Guiraud, J., Kushnerenko, E., Tomalski, P., Davies, K., Ribeiro, H., Johnson, M., & The BASIS Team, (2011). Differential habituation to repeated sounds in infants at high risk for autism. Developmental Neuroscience, DOI: 10.1097/WNR.0b013e32834c0bec.

Hadjikhani, N., Johnels, J., Zürcher, N., Lassalle, A., Guillon, Q, Hippolyte, L., & ... Gillberg, C., (2017). Look me in the eyes: constraining gaze in the eye-region provokes abnormally high subcortical activation in autism. Scientific Reports, 7:3163 | DOI:10.1038/ s41598-017-03378-5.

Hare, T., Tottenham, N., Galvan, A., Voss, H., Glover, G., & Casey, B., (2008). Biological substrates of emotional reactivity and regulation in adolescence during an emotional go-nogo task. Biol Psychiatry, 63(10):927-934, doi:10.1016/j.biopsych.2008.03.015015.

Herry C., Ciocchi S., Senn V., Demmou L., Muller C., Luthi, A., (2008) Switching on and off fear by distinct neuronal circuits. Nature 454:600–606.

Kleinhans, N., Johnson, L., Richards, T., Mahurin, R., Greenson, J., Dawson, T., & Aylward, E., (2009). Reduced neural habituation in the amygdala and social impairments in autism spectrum disorder. American Journal of Psychiatry, 166, 467-475.

Perez, J.A., Clinton, S.M., Turner, C.A., Watson, S.J., & Akin, H. (2009). A new role for FGF2 as an endogenous inhibitor of anxiety. Journal of Neuroscience, 29(19), 6379-6387.

Plieger, T., Montag, C., Felten, A., Reuter, M. (2017). The serotonin transporter polymorphism (5-HTTLPR) and personality: response style as a new endophenotype for anxiety. International Journal of Neuropsychopharmacology, 17, 6, P 851-858, https://doi.org/10.1017/S1461145713001776.

Pruessner, J.C., Dedovic, K., Pruessner, M., Lord, C., Buss, C., Collins, L., ... Lupien, S.J. (2009). Stress regulation in the central nervous system: Evidence from structural and functional neuroimaging studies in human populations. Psychoneuroendocrinology, 35(1), 179-191.

Rankin, C. Abrams, T., Barry, R., Bhatnagar, S., Clayton, D., Colombo, J., ... & Thompson, R. (2008). Habituation revisited: An updated and revised description of the behavioral characteristics of habituation. Neurobiology of Learning and Memory 92(2):135-8.

Roberts, A., Reichl, J., Song, M., Dearinger, A., Moridzadeh, N., Lu, E., ...& Glanzman, D. (2012). Habituation of the C-start response in larval zebrafish exhibits several distinct phases and sensitivity to NMDA receptor blockade. PLoS One. 2011;6(12):e29132. doi: 10.1371/journal.pone.0029132. Epub 2011 Dec 28.

Swartz, J., Wiggins, J., Carrasco, M., Lord, C., & Monk, S., (2013). Amygdala Habituation and Prefrontal Functional Connectivity in Youth With Autism Spectrum Disorders. J Am Acid Child Adolesc Psychiatry, 52(1): 84-93. doi:10.1016/j.jaac.2012.10.012.

Tam, F., King, J., Geisler, D., Korb, F., Sareng, J., Ritschel, ... Ehrlich, S., (2017). Altered behavioral and amygdale habitation in high-functioning adults with autism spectrum disorder: an fMRI study. Scientific Reports, 7:13611 | DOI:10.1038/s41598-017-14097-2.

Turk-Browne, N., Scholl, Br., & Chun, M., (2008). Babies and brains: habituation in infant cognition and functional neuroimaging. Frontiers in Human Neuroscience, doi: 10.3389/ neuro.-09.016.2008.

Webb, S., Jones, E., Merkle, K., Namkung, J., Toth, K., Greenson, J., ...Dawson, G., (2010). Toddlers With Elevated Autism Sysmptoms Show Slowed Habitation To Faces. Hild Neuropsychol, 6(3): 255-278. Doi:10.1080/09297041003601454.

Wiggins, J., Swartz, J., Martin, D., Lord, C., & Monk, C., (2014). Serotonin transporter genotype impacts amygdale habituation in youth with autism spectrum disorders. doi:10.109

CHAPTER 9 - ALLOSTATIC OVERLOAD

McEwen, B. (2005) Stressed or stressed out: What is the difference? J Psychiatry Neurosci. 2005 Sep; 30(5): 315–318.

McEwen, B. & Gianaros, P., (2010). Central role of the brain in stress and adaptation: links to socioeconomic status, health, and disease. Annals of the New York Academy of Sciences 1186 (2010) 190-222.

PART II

WHAT DIFFERENCE DOES IT MAKE?

Chapter 10
STRESS AND MORTALITY

Stress appears to shorten the lives of those with autism. Individuals with autism are reported to have an increased risk of mortality as compared with matched general population controls. On average, those with autism die 16 years earlier. The mean age of death documented for those with ASD was 53.87 years compared to individuals in the control group who died at a mean age of 70. 2 years (Hirvikoski et al., 2016).

Consistent with earlier research, a large sample of 64,637 participants found shorter leukocyte telomere length to be associated with higher mortality for all causes of death (Deelen et al., 2014; Kimura et al., 2008; Rode et al., 2015). Telomeres are nucleoprotein structures, "caps," at the ends of chromosomes that protect genomic DNA from damage during replication. Telomeres naturally shorten with age during each replication cycle until they reach a critical length, and then they no longer divide (Blackburn, 2005; Heidinger et al., 2012). The progressive shortening leads to cell aging, death, or mutation affecting the health and lifespan of an individual (Shammas, 2011). Telomere length is an independent predictor of overall cancer rate survival (Zhang et al., 2015).

There are now convergent findings across large population-based samples that psychological stress is a key contributor to accelerated telomere attrition in both children and adults (Blackburn & Epel, 2012). Highly important research investigations have uncovered that children with autism have leuko-cyte telomeres that are significantly shorter than normal (Li et al., 2014; Nelson et al., 2015).

Newborns whose mothers experienced high levels of stress during pregnancy had significantly shorter telomeres compared to newborns of mothers with low stress levels (Entringer et al., 2013; Marchetto et al., 2016; Send et al., 2016). The difference in newborn infant telomere length between high-stress and low-stress mothers was due to a shift in the telomere length distribution, with the high-stress group showing an under-representation of longer telom-eres and an over-representation of shorter telomeres (Marched et al., 2016; Send et al., 2016). In an animal study, embryos of chicks were treated with the synthetic glucocorticoid corticosterone. The newborn treated chicks had telomeres that were shorter than normal and displayed sustained reactions to an acute stressor (failure to habituate) (Haussmann et al., 2012).

Children of kindergarten age who were identified as having a combination of higher sympathetic reactivity, greater parasympathetic withdrawal, and higher cortisol response to an acute stressor had shorter buccal cell telomere lengths than their peers (Kroenke et al., 2011). Accelerated telomere attrition has been identified in children who have been exposed to stressful condi-tions. Children repeatedly exposed to the trauma of domestic violence, phys-ical abuse, and/or bullying have been found to have telomeres significantly shorter than others (Shalev et al., 2012). Children from disadvantaged social environments also have shorter-than-normal telomeres (Asok et al., 2013; Drury et al., 2012; Mitchell et al., 2014; Shalev et al., 2012). The longer children spent in a Romanian orphanage, the shorter were their telomeres (Drury et al., 2012). Social isolation in animals has also been linked to shorter telomere length. Parrots who were housed separately had significantly shorter telomeres than parrots who were housed with another bird (Aydi-nonat et al., 2014). Stressful conditions contribute to shorter telomere length, but they do not appear to account for shorter telomeres in children with autism. Poverty, neglect, and abuse are not conditions particularly associated with autism. Children with autism come from homes similar to children in the general population. Why then does autism predispose an individual to having shorter-than-normal telomeres associated with shorter life spans? More importantly, what if anything can be done about it?

Not only does stress impact the defining symptoms of autism and potentially shorten these individuals lives, it also is associated with their comorbid symptoms. Secondary symptoms that characteristically are associated with this disorder are also impacted by stress.

Chapter 11
COMORBID SYMPTOMS

The secondary comorbid symptoms of autism can be debilitating. Research findings have highlighted anxiety, gastrointestinal disorders, and tics as frequently occurring stress-related comorbid symptoms. A malfunctioning stress response can cause or exacerbate comorbid symptoms.

Anxiety. Anxiety is the most prevalent comorbid condition of autism with rates estimated between 40-80% of the population (Sukhodolsky et al., 2008). Though the terms stress and anxiety are often used interchangeably, they are separate constructs. Stress causes anxiety in both humans and laboratory animals (Griffon et al., 2007; Mitra et al., 2005; Mitra et al., 2008). A non-adaptive physiological response to stress likely contributes to the high prevalence of anxiety disorders in individuals with autism (Hollocks et al., 2014). Individuals with autism and anxiety disorders show abnormal heart rates and often blunted cortisol responses to stressors. The malfunctioning of their stress response is associated with their anxiety levels (Hollocks et al., 2014; Corbett et al., 2009). When those with autism have anxiety and social deficits that co-occur, they impact amygdala activity differently than when each occurs independently (Herrington et al., 2016).

Toddlers and older children with autism and high anxiety have significantly more repetitive behaviors, circumscribed interests, and sensory processing problems than those with low anxiety (Ben-Sasson et al., 2008; Rodgers et al., 2012). It has also been determined that anxiety is highly associated with gastrointestinal (GI) disorders (Mazurek et al., 2013).

Gastrointestinal (GI) Disorders. GI disorders including constipation, diarrhea, and abdominal discomfort occur at higher rates than normal in children with autism (Chaidez et al., 2014). GI problems are directly associated with elevated stress hormones and abnormal amygdalar activity (Myers & Greenwood-Van Meerveld, 2009). Heart rate variability, a measure of parasympathetic modulation of cardiac activity and an indicator of stress levels, was found to be positively associated with lower gastrointestinal tract symptomatology. This relationship was particularly strong for participants who had a co-occurring diagnosis of an anxiety disorder. These findings suggest there is an association between autonomic function and comorbid gastrointestinal problems in children with autism (Ferguson et al., 2017). Recall that while participating in my stress regulation program, the boy with autism who had IBS became asymptomatic. I found it fascinating that anxiety, sensory over-responsivity, and GI problems appear to be interrelated with a common biological underlying mechanism (Mazurek et al., 2013).

Tics. Another highly prevalent comorbid symptom of autism is tics. An estimated 22% of children with autism have comorbid tic disorders (Canitano et al., 2007). Individuals with tics are often diagnosed with Tourette syndrome and OCD (Huisman-van Dijk et al., 2016). Research suggests a dysregulation of stress hormones is closely linked to tics. Findings published in the journal, Neurology in February 2013, reported two boys ages six and ten were treated with fluticasone for asthma. Fluticasone is a synthetic glucocorticoid. It is administered by nasal spray and available over-the-counter. When treated with the glucocorticoid, the younger of the two children developed tics, and the tics already occurring in the older boy increased. When the physicians discontinued the medication, the tics stopped in the younger boy and returned to baseline in the older child. The same increase in tics occurred when the older boy was given the medication a second time (Steele

& Rosner, 2013). Fluticasone alters cortisol levels and research indicates children with Tourette syndrome have abnormal cortisol levels. The more extreme the abnormality in cortisol, the more severe are the tics (Corbett et al., 2008; Weiner et al., 1999). As previously mentioned, during my stress regulation program, a mother reported her son's tics had stopped.

Chapter 12
THE ORIGINS OF STRESS IN AUTISM

Problems with stress regulation can stem from sources other than neglect or trauma and can originate prior to birth. The inability to regulate stress can be: a) inherited or b) due to fetal exposure to stress hormones during the pregnancy. Under both circumstances, the fetus can be impacted without directly experiencing trauma. These two sources could account for the extreme stress of children with autism who come from loving and supportive homes. Both inherited genes and genes altered due to prenatal stress are directly connected to the stress response. Two genes, NR3C1-the glucocorticoid receptor gene (GR) and NR3C2 -the mineralocorticoid receptor (MR) are extremely important in the stress response. Alterations in these genes are found in the brains of those with autism (Patel et al., 2016; Ruzzo, 2019).

Inherited Stress. Trauma experienced by a parent or a grandparent appears capable of altering glucocorticoid receptor (GR) genes that can be passed to offspring. Males or females can transmit these genes to generations of future offspring who have not experienced trauma (Harris & Seckl, 2011; McEwen, 2012; Rodgers et al., 2013). NR3C2 has been determined to be a "heritable autism risk gene". Inherited deletions in the promoters of NR3C2 are found in those with autism. Sensory hypersensitivity occurs in individuals with deletions in NR3C2. Studies found that social problems and sleep disturbances in zebrafish occur with the loss of this gene (Ruzzo et al., 2019). Sensory hypersensitivity, social problems, and sleep disturbances are all symptoms of autism. Epigenetic modifications of NR3C1 were found in mothers exposed to trauma and in their offspring (Yehuda et al., 2014).

Prenatal Stress. According to the American Psychological Association approximately 1 in 3 women is extremely stressed; many will become pregnant. The sources of stress for pregnant women vary, but a particularly potent stressor is concern over the outcome of their pregnancy (Hompes et al., 2013; Dunkel & Tanner, 2012). With autism rates continuously climbing, pregnant women's stress has also likely escalated. Current data from the Center for Disease Control (2020) indicate 1 of 54 children are diagnosed with autism. Elevated stress hormones in a mother has consequences for the fetus. Two groups of women, one with high anxiety and the other without, were administered a mild stressor. When all mothers were stressed, the fetuses of the highly anxious women reacted; the other fetuses did not. When highly anxious pregnant women are exposed to a mild stressor, their fetuses show significant increases in heart rate (Monk et al., 2004).

Higher levels of maternal stress during pregnancy can produce abnormally elevated levels of cortisol. Prenatal stress can expose fetuses to excessive maternally derived glucocorticoids (Weinstock, 2011). Glucocorticoids are necessary for normal fetal development, but fetal exposure to elevated glucocorticoids, natural or synthetic, can alter genes that program the fetal HPA axis. The human fetal HPA axis functions at 22 weeks old (Mesiano & Jaffe, 1997). High anxiety in mothers significantly increases DNA methylation of NR3C1 in newborns (Homies et al., 2013; Oberlander et al., 2008). Infants at age 3 months with increased methylation had altered HPA axis stress reactivity and higher cortisol levels than infants with normal methylation (Oberlander et al., 2008).

Animal studies have found that these stress-related genetic alterations are sex-linked. In mice, prenatal stress very early in the pregnancy alters placental gene expression patterns differently in males than in females. In humans, males are four times more likely to have autism than females (CDC 2020). Long-term alterations in glucocorticoid receptor (GR) expression, as well as increased HPA axis responsivity, were present in prenatally stressed male mice far more frequently than in females (Mueller & Bale, 2008).

Maternal cortisol levels naturally increase during pregnancy but can become abnormally high due to stressors. The amount of fetal exposure to maternal cortisol is regulated by a placental enzyme, 11β-hydroxysteroid dehydrogenase type 2 (11β-HSD2). This enzyme regulates the flux of the glucocorticoid cortisol from the mother to the fetus. In order to protect the fetus from high concentrations of maternal cortisol, 11β-HSD2 will oxidize cortisol changing it into its less active metabolite cortisone (Murphy et al., 1974). High maternal anxiety, however, can down-regulate 11β-HSD2, allowing maternal stress hormones freer access to the fetus. Inhibition of the fetal-placental barrier to maternal glucocorticoids in rats causes an increase in glucocorticoid receptor mRNA in the basolateral amygdala and increases anxiety-like behavior (Welberg, 2001). In rats exposed to prenatal stress, there was an increase of 30% in overall brain volume and an accompanying increase in neurons of 49% (Salm et al., 2004). Increases in brain volume, as previously noted, also occur with autism.

The reprogramming of the HPA axis of the fetus causes future problems with stress regulation and alterations in genes (Huizink et al., 2004; Molteni et al., 2001; Mueller & Bale 2008; Sandman, 2011; Shoener et al., 2006). Greater prenatal stress is associated with a failure to habituate. This inability to get used to things was previously discussed as a characteristic feature of the malfunctioning stress response in those with autism. In a recent study, cortisol and stress levels were assessed in mothers during their third trimester of pregnancy. When the offspring turned nine-months-old, they were exposed to a repeated experimental stressor, separation from their mother. The babies were divided into two groups-those from anxious mothers and those from mothers who were not. All infants were temporarily removed from their mothers on three separate occasions. After the first separation, the cortisol levels returned to normal in the infants of low stress mothers indicating habituation. Infants born from mothers reporting high levels of stress during the pregnancy, however, were significantly less likely to habituate to the experimental separation. They cried and fussed more during the first separation. Their cortisol levels remained elevated for all three sessions indicating an active stress response throughout. Interestingly, the crying decreased in both groups upon repeated separations, but cortisol levels remained high in the group whose mothers were anxious. Although overt signs of stress may diminish, it should not be assumed that the stress response has terminated. These infants were still experiencing stress, but no longer crying for help (de Weerth et al., 2015).

Chapter 13
STRESS AT BIRTH

One might speculate that if individuals with autism were impacted by inherited genes or prenatal stress, then evidence of a malfunctioning stress response would be present at birth, and indeed, it is. The impact of stress on telomeres and habituation have been previously discussed. In addition to shorter telomeres and an inability to habituate, atypical crying and abnormal pupillary light reflex (PLR) are also signs of an abnormal stress response. All are evident in those more likely to later be diagnosed with autism.

High frequency cries (above 1 kHz) have been linked to poor regulation of the stress response and autism. There is a significant association between NR3C1 methylation and the presence of very high fundamental frequencies in cry utterances in infants (Reggiannini et al., 2013; Sheinkopf et al., 2012). Crying is vital for infant survival. Crying can serve to recruit a caregiver to restore balance to an infant's system under stress. Vocal recordings of cries from 6-month-old infants who were at higher risk for autism (ASD; n = 21) and the cries of low-risk infants (n = 18) were compared. Cries were categorized by acoustic analyses as either pain-related or non-pain-related. Infants at greater risk produced pain-related cries with higher and more variable fundamental frequency than low-risk infants. At-risk infants later diagnosed with autism at 36 months had among the highest values (Sheinkopf et al., 2012).

Caretakers react differently to higher frequency cries (Esposito & Vent, 2009). Adults, both female and male, react differently to the cries of infants later diagnosed with autism than to those of neurotypical infants. The higher frequency cries are said to be more difficult to interpret and in general elicit negative feelings in adults. Different brain regions than normal are activated in adults in response to infants' higher frequency cries. The autonomic nervous system of male adults listening to recorded cries of infants who later were diagnosed with autism responded with greater galvanic skin responses and more emotional arousal than when those men listened to cries of neurotypical infants (Esposito et al., 2015). Adults behave differently when attempting to soothe an infant with higher frequency cries (Apicella et al., 2013; Esposito et al., 2015; Esposito et al., 2017). This signature characteristic of high frequency cries could assist in identifying neonates who are at greater risk for later being diagnosed with autism.

In addition to higher frequency crying, further evidence of a malfunctioning stress response in infants can be detected by examining the baby's eyes. The pupillary light reflex (PLR) reacts to stressors both physical and psychological (Davis et al., 2013). Reactions of the pupil are modulated by the parasympathetic system and are a reliable measure of parasympathetic dysfunction (Wang et al., 2016). Those with autism have an abnormal PLR and, as previously reported, parasympathetic dysfunction. The magnitude of the pupil's constriction in response to changes in light in infancy is associated with a diagnosis of autism at 3 years old and predicts symptom severity (Nyström et al., 2018). As noted earlier, the degree of sensory dysfunction is significantly correlated with decreased PLR constriction amplitude (Daluwatte et al., 2015).

The problems with regulating stress during infancy continue into early childhood and are further complicated by a variety of environmental stressors. At very early ages the majority of toddlers and preschoolers navigate in dynamic, challenging social environments without their parents (Watamura et al., 2003). Children attending daycare programs (that were not in a home setting) had higher cortisol levels according to nine different studies than those at home or in home daycares. Even children who attend day care settings that have been given high-quality ratings demonstrate a rise rather than the healthy decline in cortisol throughout the day. In one high-quality daycare setting, 91% of the children displayed irregular cortisol rhythms. Conversely, children cared for in the home environments of others show the predictable normal decline in cortisol following the morning peak (Watamura et al. 2002). The most marked elevations in cortisol were found in those between the ages of two and three. The toddlers with the poorer social skills had the higher stress levels. Toddlers with autism show significantly more severe early signs of avoidance of others in social interactions and are more anxious than typical children (Davis III et al., 2009; Vermeer & IJzendoorn, 2006).

Once signs of excessive stress are identified, treatment efforts need to begin. The remainder of the book addresses stress in those with autism from two different perspectives. The first addresses their stress directly offering treatment in individual or in small groups settings. The second focuses on prevention and addresses stress that effects those with autism from a more global perspective within the general population.

REFERENCES

CHAPTER 10 - STRESS AND MORTALITY

Asok, A., Bernard, K., Roth, T., Rosen, J., & Dozier, M., (2013). Parental Responsiveness Moderates the Association Between Early-life Stress and Reduced Telomere Length. DevPsychopathol, 25(3): 577-584.doi:10.1017/S0954579413000011.

Aydinonat, D., Penn, D., Smith, S., Moodley, Y., Hoelzl, F., Knauer, F., & Schwarzenberger, F. (2014). Social isolation shortens telomeres in African Grey parrots (Psittacus erithacus erithacus). Plos One, 9(4), e93839. doi:10.1371/journal.pone.0093839

Blackburn, E. H. (2005). Telomeres and telomerase: their mechanisms of action and the effects of altering their functions. FEBS Letters, 579(4), 859-862.

Blackburn, E. H., & Epel, E. S. (2012). Telomeres and adversity: Too toxic to ignore. Nature, 490 (7419), 169-171.

Deelen, J., Beekman, M., Cold, V., Trompet, S., Broer, L., Hägg, S., ... Slagboom, P. E. (2014). Leukocyte telomere length associates with prospective mortality independent of immune-related parameters and known genetic markers. International Journal Of Epidemiology, 43(3), 878-886. doi:10.1093/ije/dyt267.

Drury, S., Theall, K., Gleason, M., Smyke, A.., De Vivo, I., Wong, J. ., ... Nelson, C. (2012). Telomere length and early severe social deprivation: Linking early adversity and cellular aging. Molecular Psychiatry, 17(7), 719-727. doi:10.1038/mp.2011.53.

Entringer, S., Epel, E., Lin, J., Buss, C., Shahbaba, B., Blackburn, E.,& ... Wadhwa, P. (2013). Maternal psychosocial stress during pregnancy is associated with newborn leukocyte telomere length. American Journal of Obstetrics and Gynecology, 208(2), 134.e1-7. doi:10.1016/j.ajog.2012.11.033.

Haussmann, M. F., Longenecker, A. S., Marchetto, N. M., Juliano, S. A., & Bowden, R. M. (2012). Embryonic exposure to corticosterone modifies the juvenile stress response, oxidative stress and telomere length. Proceedings. Biological Sciences / The Royal Society, 279(1732), 1447-1456. doi:10.1098/rspb.2011.1913.

Heidinger, B. J., Blount, J. D., Boner, W., Griffiths, K., Metcalfe, N. B., & Monaghan, P. (2012). Telomere length in early life predicts lifespan. Proceedings of the National Academy of Sciences of the United States of America, 109(5), 1743-1748. doi:10.1073/pnas.1113306109.

Hirvikoski, T., Mittendorfer-Rutz, E., Boman, M., Larsson, H., Lichtenstein, P., & Bölte, S. (2016). Premature mortality in autism spectrum disorder. The British Journal of Psychiatry, 1-7.doi:10.1192bjp.bp.114.160192.

Kimura, M., Cherkas, L. F., Kato, B. S., Demissie, S., Hjelmborg, J. B., Brimacombe, M., ... Aviv, A. (2008). Offspring's leukocyte telomere length, paternal age, and telomere elongation in sperm. Plos Genetics, 4(2), e37. doi:10.1371/journal.pgen.0040037.

Kroenke, C. H., Epel, E., Adler, N., Bush, N. R., Obradovic, J., Lin, J., ... Boyce, W. T. (2011). Autonomic and adrenocortical reactivity and buccal cell telomere length in kindergarten children. Psychosomatic Medicine, 73(7), 533-540. doi:10.1097/PSY.0b013e318229acfc.

Li, Z., Tang, J., Li, H., Chen, S., He, Y., Liao, Y., ... Chen, X. (2014). Shorter telomere length in peripheral blood leukocytes is associated with childhood ASD. Scientific Reports, 47073. doi:10.1038/srep07073.

Marchetto, N., Glynn, R., Ferry, M., Ostojic, M., Wolff, S., Yao, R. & Haussmann, M. (2016). Prenatal stress and newborn telomere length. Am J Obstet Gynecol. 2016 Jul;215(1):94.e1-8. doi: 10.1016/j.ajog.2016.01.177. Epub 2016 Jan 30.

Mitchell, C., Hobcraft, J., McLanahan, S., Siegel, S., Berg, A., Brooks-Gunn, j., & ... Notterman,D., (2014). Social disadvantage, genetic sensitivity, and children's telomere length. ProcNatl Acad Sci, 111(16):5944-9. doi:10.1073/pnas.140429311.

Nelson, C. A., Varcin, K. J., Coman, N. K., DeVivo, I., & Tager-Flusberg, H. (2015). Shortened Telomeres in Families with a Propensity to ASD. Journal of the American Academy Of Child And Adolescent Psychiatry, 54(7),588-594. doi:10.1016/j.jaac.2015.04.006.

Rode, L., Nordestgaard, B. G., & Bojesen, S. E. (2015). Peripheral blood leukocyte telomere length and mortality among 64,637 individuals from the general population. Journal of the National Cancer Institute, 107(6), djv074. doi:10.1093/jnci/djv074.

Send, T., Gilles, M., Codd, V., Wolf, I., Bardtke, S., Streit, F., ...& Witt, S. (2017). Telomere Length in Newborns is Related to Maternal Stress During Pregnancy. Neuropsychopharmacology. 2017 Nov;42(12):2407-2413. doi: 10.1038/npp.2017.73.

Shalev, I., Moffitt, T. E., Sugden, K., Williams, B., Houts, R. M., Danese, A., ... Caspi, A. (2012). Exposure to violence during childhood is associated with telomere erosion from 5 to 10 years of age: a longitudinal study. Molecular Psychiatry, 18(5), 576-581. doi:10.1038/mp.2012.32.

Shammas, M. A., (2011)Telomeres, lifestyle, cancer, and ageing. Current Opinion in Clinical Nutritional Metabolic Care, 14(1): 28-34. doi:10.1097/MCO/Ob013e32834121b1.

Zhang, C., Chen, X., Li, L., Zhou, Y., Wang, C., Hou, S., (2015) The association between telomere length and cancer prognosis: evidence from a meta-analysis. PLoS ONE, 10(7):e0133174.doi:10.1371/journal.pone.0133174.

CHAPTER 11 - COMORBID SYMPTOMS

Ben-Sasson, A., Cermak, S., Orsmond, G., Tager-Flusberg, H., Kadlec, M., & Carter, A., (2008). Sensory clusters of toddlers with autism spectrum disorders: differences in affective symptoms. The Journal of Child Psychology and Psychiatry, 49:817-825.

Canitano, R., & Viventi, G. (2007). The relationship between tics, OC, ADHD and autism symptoms: A cross- disorder symptom analysis in Gilles de la Tourette syndrome patients and family-members. Pub Med https://doi.org/10.1177/1362361307070992.

Chaidez, V., Hansen, R., & Hertz-Picciotto, I. (2014) Gastrointestinal problems in children with autism, developmental delays or typical development. Autism Dev Disord. 2014 May;44(5):1117-27. doi: 10.1007/s10803-013-1973-x.

Corbett, B., Schupp, C., Levine, S., & Mendoza, S. (2009). Comparing cortisol, stress, and sensory sensitivity in children with autism. Autism Research, 2(1), 39-49.

Corbett, B.A., Mendoza, S.P., Baym, C.L., Bunge, S.A., & Levine, S. (2008). Examiningcortisol rhythmicity and responsivity to stress in children with Tourette syndrome. Psychoneuroendocrinology, 33(6), 810-820.

Ferguson, B., Marler, S., Altstein, L., Lee, E., Akers, J., Sohl, K., ...& Beiersdorf, D. (2017) Psychophysiological associations with gastrointestinal symptomatology in Autism Spectrum Disorder. Autism Res. 2017 Feb;10(2):276-288. dos: 10.1002/aur.1646. Epub 2016 Jun 20.

Griffon, C., Duncko, R., Covington, M., Kopperman, L., & Kling, M., (2007). Acute stress potentiates anxiety in humans. Biological Psychiatry, 62, 1183-1186.

Herrington, J., Miller, J., Pandey, J., Schultz, R. (2016) Anxiety and social deficits have distinct relationships with amygdala function in autism spectrum disorder. Soc Cogn Affect Neurosci. 2016 Jun;11(6):907-14. doi: 10.1093/scan/nsw015. Epub 2016 Feb 9.

Hollocks, M., Howlin, P., Papadopoulos, A., Khondoker, M., & Simonoff, E., (2014).Differences in HPA-axis and heart rate responsiveness to psychosocial stress in children with autism spectrum disorders with and without co-morbid anxiety. Psychoneuroendocrinotology, doi:101016.jpsyneuen.2014.04.004.

Huisman-van Dijk, H., Schoot, R., Rijkeboer, M., Mathews, C., & Cath, D. (2016). The relationship between tics, OC, ADHD and autism symptoms: A cross- disorder symptom analysis in Gilles de la Tourette syndrome patients and family-members. Psychiatry Res. 2016 Mar 30;237:138-46. doi: 10.1016/j.psychres.2016.01.051. Epub 2016 Jan 22.

Mazurek, M., Vasa, R., Kalb, L., Kanne, S., Rosenberg, D., Keefer, A., ... & Lowery, L. (2013). Anxiety, sensory over-responsivity, and gastrointestinal problems in children with Autism Spectrum Disorders. Journal of Abnormal Child Psychology, 41, 165-176 doi 10.1007/s10802-012-9668-x.

Mitra, R., & Sapolsky, R. (2008). Acute corticosterone treatment is sufficient to induce anxiety and amygdaloid dendritic hypertrophy. Proceedings of the National Academy of Sciences, 105(14), 5573-5578.

Mitra, R., Jadhav, S., McEwen, B., Vyas, A., & Chattarji, S., (2005). Stress duration modulates the spatiotemporal patterns of spine formation in the basolateral amygdala. Proceedings of the National Academy of Sciences of the United States of America, 102, 9371-9376. doi/10.1073/pnas.0504011102.

Myers, B., & Greenwood-Van Meerveld, B. (2009). Role of anxiety in the pathophysiology of irritable bowel syndrome. Frontiers in Enteric Neuroscience, 3(47), 1-10.

Rodgers, J., Glod, M., Connolly, B., & McConachie, H. (2012). The relationship between anxiety and repetitive behaviours in autism spectrum disorder. Journal of Autism and Developmental Disorders, 42:2404-2409.

Steele, M. & Rosner, J., (2013). A possible association between fluticasone propionate and tics in pediatric asthmatic patients: two case reports and a literature review. Neurology, 80: P0264 (meeting abstracts).

Sukhodolsky, D., Scahill, L., Gadow, K., Arnold, L., Aman, M., et al., (2008). Parent-rated anxiety symptoms in children with pervasive developmental disorders: frequency and association with core autism symptoms and cognitive functioning. Journal of Abnormal Child Psychology, 36(1), 117-128.

Weiner, P., Berar-Yanay, N., Davidovich, A., & Magadle, R. (1999). Nocturnal cortisol secretion in asthmatic patients after inhalation of fluticasone propionate. Chest. 1999 Oct;116(4):931-4.

CHAPTER 12 - THE ORIGINS OF STRESS IN AUTISM

de Weerth, C., Buitelaar, J., Beijers, R. (2015). Infant cortisol and behavioral habituation to weekly maternal separations: links with maternal prenatal cortisol and psychosocial stress. Psychoneuroendocrinology. 2013 Dec;38(12):2863-74. doi: 10.1016/j.psyneuen.2013.07.014. Epub 2013 Oct 6.

Dunked Schetter, C., & Tanner, L. (2012). Anxiety, depression and stress in pregnancy: implications for mothers, children, research, and practice. Current opinion in psychiatry, 25(2), 141–148. https://doi.org/10.1097/YCO.0b013e3283503680

Harris, A. & Seckl J., (2011). Glucocorticoids, prenatal stress and the programming of disease. Hormones and Behavior, 59, 279-289.

Hompes, T., Izzi, B., Gellens, E., Morreels, M., Fieuws, S., Pexsters, A., & ... Claes, S., (2013). Investigating the influence of maternal cortisol and emotional state during pregnancy on the DNA methylation status of the glucocorticoid receptor gene (NR3C1) promoter region in cord blood. Journal of Psychiatric Research, doi:10.1016/j.jpsychires2013.03.009.

Huizink, A, M ulder, E., & Buitelaar, J.(2004). Prenatal stress and risk for psychopathology: Specific effects or induction of general susceptibility? Psychological Bulletin, 130(1), 115-142.

McEwen, B. (2012). Brain on stress: How the social environment gets under the skin. PNAS, doi/10.1073.

Mesiano S, & Jaffe R.,1997. Developmental and functional biology of the primate fetal adrenal cortex. Endocr Rev 18:378–403.

Molteni, R., Fumagalli, F., Magnaghi, V., Roceri, M., Generally, M., Racagni, G., ... Riva, M. (2001). Modulation of FGF-2 by stress and corticosteroids: From developmental events to adult brain plasticity. Brain Research Reviews, 37(1-3), 249-258.

Monk C., Myers, M., Sloan, R., Werner, L., Jeon, J, Tager, F., & Fifer, W. (2004). Fetal heart rate reactivity differs by women's psychiatric status: an early marker for developmental risk? Journal of the American Academy of Child and Adolescent Psychiatry. 43:283–290.

Mueller, B., & Bale, T.(2008). Sex-specific programming of offspring emotionality following stress early in pregnancy. Journal of Neuroscience, 28(36), 9055-9065.

Murphy B, Clark S, Donald I, Pinsky M, & Velady D. (1974). Conversion of maternal cortisol to cortisone during placental transfer to the human fetus. Am J Obstet Gynecol; 118:538-41; PMID:4812574

Oberlander, T., Weinberg, J., Papsdorf, M., Grunau, R., Misri, S., & Devlin, A., (2008). Prenatal exposure to maternal depression, neonatal methylation of human glucocorticoid receptor gene (NR3C1) and infant cortisol stress responses. Epigenetics, 3:2, 97-106.

Patel, N., Crider, A., Pandya, C., Ahmed, A., & Pillai, A. (2016). Altered mRNA Levels of Glucocorticoid Receptor, Mineralocorticoid Receptor, and Co-Chaperones (FKBP5 and PTGES3) in the Middle Frontal Gyrus of Autism Spectrum Disorder Subjects. Mol Neurobiol 53(4):2090-9. doi:10.1007/s12035-35-015-9178-2.

Rodgers, A., Morgan, C., Bronson, S., Revello, S., & Bale, T., (2013). Paternal stress exposure alters sperm microRNA content and reprograms offspring HPA stress axis regulation. Journal of Neuroscience, 33(21):9003-9012. doi:10.1523/JNEUROSCI.0914-13.2013.

Ruzzo, E., Perez-Cano, L., Jung, J., Wang, L., Kashef-Haghigi, D. (2019). Inherited and De Novo Genetic Risk for Autism Impacts Shared Networks. Cell 178, 850-866.

Salm, A.K., Pavelko, M., Krouse, E.M., Webster, W., Kraszpulski, M., & Birkle, D.L. (2004). Lateral amygdaloid nucleus expansion in adult rats is associated with exposure to prenatal stress. Developmental Brain Research, 148(2), 159-167.

Sandman, C., Davis, E., Buss, C., & Glynna, L. (2011) Exposure to prenatal psychobiological stress exerts programming influences on the mother and her fetus. Neuroendocrinology.

Shoener, J., Baig, R., & Page, K. (2006). Prenatal exposure to dexamethasone alters hippocampal drive on hypothalamic-pituitary-adrenal axis activity in adult male rats. American Journal of Physiology -Regulatory Integrative Comparative Physiology, 290(5), R1366-1373.

Weinstock M (2011) Sex-dependent changes induced by prenatal stress in cortical and hippocampal morphology and behaviour in rats: an update. Stress 14:604–613.

Welberg, L., Secki, J., & Holmes, M. (2001). Inhibition of 11⊠-hydroxysteroid dehydrogenase, the foeto-placental barrier to maternal glucocorticoids, permanently programs amygdala GR mRNA expression and anxiety-like behavior in the offspring. European Journal of Neuroscience, 12(3), 1047-1054.

Yehuda, R., Daskalakis, N., Lehrner, A., Desarnaud, F., Bader, H., Makotkine, I., ... Meaney, M. (2014). Influences of maternal and paternal PTSD on epigenetic regulation of the glucocorticoid receptor gene in Holocaust survivor offspring. The American Journal of Psychiatry, 171(8), 872-880. doi:10.1176/appi.ajp.2014.13121571.

CHAPTER 13 . STRESS AT BIRTH

Apicella, F., Chericoni, N., Costanzo, V., Baldini, S., Billeci, L., Cohen, D., & Muratori, F. (2013). Reciprocity in interaction: a window on the first year of life in ASD. Autism Spectrum Disorder Research and Treatment, 2013705895. doi:10.1155/2013/705895.

Daluwatte, C., Miles, J., Sun, J., & Yao, G. (2015). Association between pupillary light reflex and sensory behaviors in children with autism spectrum disorders. ResDev Disabil. Feb; 37: 209-215. dos:10.1016/jridd.2014.11.019

Davis III, T., Fodstad, J., Jenkins, W., Hess, J., Moree, B., Dempsey, T., & Matson, J. (2009). Anxiety and avoidance in infants and toddlers with autism spectrum disorders: Evidence for differing symptom severity and presentation. Research in Autism Spectrum Disorders, 4(2), 305-313.

Davis, B., Daluwatte, N. Colona, N., & Yao, D. (2013) Effects of cold-pressor and mental arithmetic on pupillary light reflex. Physiological Measurement, Volume 34, Number 8.

Esposito G, Valenzi S, Islam T, Bornstein, M. (2015) Three physiological responses in fathers and non-fathers' to vocalizations of typically developing infants and infants with Autism Spectrum Disorder. Res Dev Disabil 43–44:43–50.

Esposito, G & Venuti, P. (2009) Comparative analysis of crying in children with autism, developmental delays, and typical development. Focus on Autism and Other Developmental Disabilities. https://doi.org/10.1177/1088357609336449

Esposito, G. Hiroi, N., & Scattoni, M. (2017). Cry, baby, cry: expression of distress as a biomarker and modulator in Autism Spectrum Disorder. International Journal of Neuropsychopharmacology, 20,6, 403-498-503. https://doi.org/10.1093/ijnp/pyx014.

Nyström, P., Gliga,T., Nilsson Jobs, E., Gredebäck, G., Charman, T., Johnson, M., ... & Terje Falck-Ytter, T. (2018). Enhanced pupillary light reflex in infancy is associated with autism diagnosis in toddlerhood. Nature Communications volume 9: 1678. DOI:

10.1038/s41467-018-03985-4 Open.

Reggiannini B., Sheinkopf S. J., Silverman H. F., Li X., Lester B. (2013). A flexible analysis tool for the quantitative acoustic assessment of infant cry. J. Speech Lang. Hear. Res. 56, 1416–1428. 10.1044/1092-4388(2013/11-0298).

Sheinkopf, S., Iverson, J., Rinaldi, M., & Lester, B., (2012). Atypical cry acoustics in 6 month-old infants at risk for Autism Spectrum Disorder. Autism Research, 5(5): 331-339. doi:10.1002/aur.1244.

Vermeer, H.J., & Van IJzendoorn, M.H. (2006). Children's elevated cortisol levels at daycare: A review and meta-analysis. Early Childhood Research Quarterly, 21(3), 390-401.

Wang, Y., Zkveld, A., Naylor, G., Ohlenforst, B., Jansma, E., Lorens, A., …& Kramer, S. (2016). Parasympathetic nervous system dysfunction, as identified by pupil light reflex, and its possible connection to hearing impairment. PLoS One. 2016; 11(4): e0153566. doi: 10.1371/journal.pone.0153566

Watamura, S. E., Sebanc, A. M., & Gunnar, M. R. (2002). Rising cortisol at childcare: relations with nap, rest, and temperament. Developmental psychobiology, 40(1), 33–42. https://doi.org/10.1002/dev.1001

Watamura, S.E., Donzella, B., Alain, J., & Gunnar, M.R. (2003). Morning-to-afternoon increases in cortisol concentrations for infants and toddlers at child care: Age differences and behavioral correlates. Child Development, 74(4), 1006-1020.

PART III

WHAT CAN BE DONE ABOUT IT?

Chapter 14
BENEFITS OF TREATMENT

Treatment and prevention efforts can improve symptoms and may extend the lives of children with autism. Direct evidence documents the benefits of stress regulation. Treatments have been shown to a) decrease brain volume (Hölzel et al., 2010); b) favorably modify gene expression (Bhasin et al., 2013, Dusek et al., 2008); and c) improve operations of the ANS and HPA axis (Esch et al., 2003; Manzoni et al., 2008; Tang et al., 2007). Fortunately, brain plasticity can be promoted, telomeres can be lengthened, and glucocorticoids better regulated. The highlights of key investigations follow.

Brain plasticity. After eight weeks of a mindfulness-based intervention, participants who were highly anxious showed significant decreases in right basolateral amygdala gray matter density and reported significantly less stress. The greater the decrease in stress, the greater was the decrease in amygdaloid gray matter density (Hölzel et al., 2010). This is particularly germane to children with autism due to their abnormal amygdalar volumes and high anxiety. As previously noted, amygdalar volume in children with autism can be as much as 16% larger than normal by age 2 (Mosconi et al., 2009). Anxiety is the most prevalent comorbid condition of autism and is positively correlated with increased amygdalar volume in children with autism. The excessive growth of the amygdala in a child with autism might be halted or reversed through stress regulation. The outdated notion that brain structure does not change has been replaced with physical evidence that the brain is highly plastic (Kolb & Gibb, 2011; McEwen & Morrison, 2013).

As previously discussed, the dendrites of the soil nematode Caenorhabditis elegans increased and returned to normal based on stress exposure. Neurons in rat brains altered by stress also returned to normal after the stressor was removed; brain plasticity was found to be age-dependent: the younger the rat, the greater its recovery (Bloss et al., 2010; Radley et al., 2005).

Gene Expression. Genes do not have to dictate a child's destiny. Brain development reflects more than the simple unfolding of an inherited genetic blueprint; it is shaped by a complex interaction of both healthy and unhealthy genetic and experiential factors (Kolb & Gibb, 2011). Genetic analysis revealed that after only one session of meditation, novice practitioners showed epigenetic changes in the direction that would benefit stress regulation and the immune response. Long-term practitioners had far more transcriptional changes than beginners, but there were overlapping patterns between the two groups. Changes persisted outside of the sessions for both groups (Bhasin et al., 2013). Another study found further evidence of epigenetic changes from treatment after eight weeks of mindfulness training. Participants newly trained in mindfulness techniques showed significant, long-term changes in cellular metabolism after eight weeks. Gene expression profiles found that 1,561 genes were differentially expressed in this group of participants compared to the control. Epigenetic changes also overlapped with long-term practitioners, again suggesting sustainability. Gene analysis indicated that the changes could likely counteract cellular damage related to chronic psychological stress. The study was successfully replicated (Dusek et al., 2008).

The accelerated shortening of telomeres, which is associated with shorter life spans and disease, appears to be preventable. As previously noted, children with autism have significantly shorter telomeres. In the group of children with autism, only those who had participated in a "family training interven-

tion" had significantly longer leukocyte telomeres than those who did not
(Li et al., 2014). Among high-risk children, those who received dedicated
maternal care had longer telomeres (Asok et al., 2014).

Increased activity levels of the enzyme telomerase can lengthen telomeres
(Blackburn, 2000). Telomerase facilitates the addition of DNA sequences
which elongate telomeres (Armanios & Blackburn, 2012; Blackburn, 2010;
Kim et al., 2003). Interventions that target stress have been shown to increase
telomerase activity. Mindfulness meditation leads to increased telomerase
activity in peripheral blood mononuclear cells (Schutte & Malouff, 2014).
Increased telomerase activity is associated with decreased levels of chronic
stress, lower cortisol, and less anxiety (Daubenmier et al., 2012).

ANS and the HPA axis. Evidence indicates regulating stress can impact both
the ANS and the HPA axis. Regulating stress decreases sympathetic nervous
system activity and increases parasympathetic activity, important in relaxation. Cortisol also decreases when stress is better regulated (Esch et al.,
2003; Manzoni et al., 2008; Tang et al., 2007). Tai chi has demonstrated
consistent and significant efficacy in lowering the heart rate, decreasing cortisol, and reducing anxiety. The benefits are documented in a meta-analysis
of 36 studies with 3,799 adult participants (Rogers et al., 2009). Tai chi was
used as the primary meditative exercise in my feasibility studies.

Chapter 15
TREATING CHILDREN WITH AUTISM - FEASIBILITY STUDIES

A feasibility study is research conducted to see if something can be done. The purpose of my two feasibility studies was to determine if meditative interventions that have been shown to promote relaxation in adults could be adapted to accommodate children with autism and other neurodevelopmental disabilities. Meditative exercises are done quietly with stillness and focus. This raises the question of feasibility when attempting to train children to relax, particularly with those who have short attention spans and endless energy. Based on sound psychological principles and years of professional experience, I successfully designed and implemented such a program. All but one of twenty-four participants, ages 6 through 12, with ASD, TS, and ADHD, demonstrated they could participate in the stress regulation program. (One of the younger children could not tolerate being separated from his father.) Attendance in both studies averaged over 90%. Videotapes, observations, and written feedback documented that the trainers had conducted the program with fidelity. Not only could the children participate, but data indicate they reaped significant physical and psychosocial benefits. Parents and teachers reported that the documented improvements generalized to home and school, attesting to the intervention's social validity.

Group Dynamics. In addition to meditative exercises, self-control, and leadership were promoted. At the beginning of each session, participants took turns standing and answering a simple question (e.g., "what is your favorite food?"). Initially, interruptions of the speaker were discouraged by the trainers, but as the program progressed participants monitored each other. During each session, all participants were given turns to lead group activities; some required more guidance in their leadership roles than others.

Clinically, children were provided with instructions on addressing stressors at home and in school. Each session began with group dialogue.

Quantitative Data. Significant results were obtained from data collected with the following standardized instruments: the Behavior Rating Inventory for Executive Functioning (BRIEF), the ACTeRS Behavior Rating Scale, the Conners' Parent Rating Scales-Revised Short Form and the Revised Children's Manifest Anxiety Scale (session two). An alpha level of .05 was set for probability levels of all assessments. The extent of improvements documented by these measures was far greater than expected.

The BRIEF assesses executive functioning within eight derived clinical scales. The executive functions are processes responsible for guiding, directing, and managing cognition, emotion, and behavior. The eight clinical scales combine to form the Global Executive Composite (GEC) which is designed to measure the overall ability to perform executive functions. After the first feasibility study, results from the BRIEF indicated that the mean improvement on the GEC was 1.5 standard deviations (SD), and each of the eight clinical executive functioning scales increased more than 1 SD.

The ACTeRS monitors the effects of intervention on the behavioral categories of: Attention, Hyperactivity, Social Skills, and Oppositional Behavior. The results from the first study indicated significant improvements in three areas: attention, hyperactivity, and socialization.

The Conners' Parent Rating Scales-Revised Short Form incorporates four subscales: Oppositional, Cognitive Problems, Hyperactivity, and ADHD Index. The Conners' Global Index (CGI) consists of 10 items that have been determined to be the most sensitive to treatment effects. This instrument provides information on hyperactivity, inattentiveness, and a tendency for pronounced emotional reaction. Results from the first study indicated that three of the six participants improved > 2 SDs and no longer scored in the "Indicates Significant Problem" range on the CGI.

The Revised Children's Manifest Anxiety Scale is a 49 item self-reporting measure that assesses the nature and levels of anxiety in participants from 6-19 years-of-age. The instrument yields six scales: Defensiveness, Inconsistent Responding, Total Anxiety, Physiological Anxiety, Worry, and Social Anxiety. This was administered only for the second study. Findings from the children's responses overall were statistically significant, including the subclasses: Worry and Physiological Anxiety.

Many areas in the second study indicated improvement but did not reach significance. Children met twice weekly in the first study and only one time a week in the second study. This was likely a contributing factor to the results.

Qualitative Data. Qualitative data were gathered from: the participants, their parents and teachers. Data was gathered before and after each session from the children and pre- and post-intervention from the parents.

The participants provided written feedback and reported "tai chi is fun" 76% of the time. They consistently rated on an examiner developed test that they feel more like a horse-drawn buggy than a race car at the end of the sessions. The children expressed disappointment and a desire for the program to continue when told it would be ending.

Input from parents was submitted on a program summary form and obtained during individual interviews. Their comments have been interjected throughout the book. Those not previously mentioned include observed improvements in self-image and social skills. The mother of the child with TS indicated that her son's self-esteem had "suffered so much from embarrassing tics. Tai chi helped him feel really good about himself." Another parent remarked, "Tai chi is great for a child; it gives him a feeling of self-worth!"

The participants were also described as being more socially engaged and considerate. For example, one mother of a boy with ASD shared this anecdote:

In the middle of December we attended a mother-son dance. To begin with, my son actually wanted to go to the dance, and this was pretty incredible by itself. We had so much fun that night. He danced, sang, and really enjoyed himself. He encouraged other children to dance and asked other mothers to dance.

I am a fervent believer in rigorous research and relied upon it for the foundation and substance of this book. In critiquing the work, it is important to keep in mind that this research was conducted as feasibility studies -never intended to be randomized controlled trials. There is substantial data to support that the children were able to participate in the program.

The data for measuring progress, however, should be interpreted more cautiously. One should differentiate and exercise caution when assessing progress based on the data for a number of reasons including the small sample size and uncontrolled variables. Future studies should include larger more representative samples; fewer external variables; and control groups. Even though these studies had obvious weaknesses they were capable of being replicated with different trainers and data collection was conducted with key elements in place. Both studies used: a) qualitative and quantitative data; b) data obtained from psychometric instruments that were standardized on large populations; and c) multiple sources of data input.

A teacher candidly expressed her initial doubts and subsequent approval. She remarked after the sessions concluded, "I was a skeptic. I didn't believe tai chi would help, but I saw it happen. I didn't think it would make a difference, but it did." Children of school age can be taught to minimize stressors and trained in methods to relax.

Chapter 16
TREATMENT MODEL

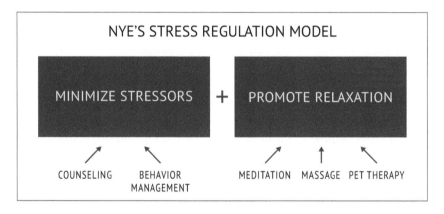

I developed a treatment model based on the feasibility studies and subsequent research. The model is built on sound psychological principles, revolutionary findings in neuroscience, and the time-tested practices of Eastern medicine. The model was specifically designed for those with autism of all ages, but can be used with a range of disabilities. It is well suited for broad scale application in public and private schools, hospitals, and clinics.

The model proposes a primary goal of improved stress regulation. The method involves a two-pronged approach for regulating stress: minimize stressors and promote relaxation. Both should be addressed simultaneously. The model specifically targets stress generated by sensory stimuli and social interactions. There needs to be fewer, less potent stressors and individuals need to be trained to better relax. The intervention can be utilized with individuals or in small groups. Group size largely depends on age and functioning levels. An assistant is always recommended.

Psychological counseling is critical in the delivery of services. Counseling is needed to assist in both minimizing stressors and promoting relaxation. The counselor can provide leadership in coordinating the efforts of other critical personnel and family members. Children with autism (and their parents) are entitled to psychological counseling services under federal law as detailed in Section 300.34 of the Individuals with Disabilities Education Act (IDEA). Children need to be better prepared for addressing stressors, and this is particularly true for those with autism. For guidance in delivering the services, a "best practices" manual for addressing stress in those with autism would be beneficial. The effort would likely be most fruitful if developed by a team of experts from across disciplines including physicians, psychologists, school administrators, counselors, occupational therapists, and behavioral therapists.

Clinical interventions. Control and leadership are key clinical elements in regulating stress. There is likely overlap but each plays an important role.

Stressors are perceived as far less severe if an individual or animal feels in control of the stressor. For the same external stressor, subjects feel less subjectively stressed, activate less of a stress response, and are less at risk for a stress-related disease if they feel a sense of control (Karasak, 1979). It follows that clinical support to train children with autism in methods to acquire and maintain self-control would empower them. Self-control can assist in minimizing stressors and in training methods for relaxation.

As a regular part of my program, exercises were practiced to train children to exercise self-control. One such exercise encouraged children to stand still silently. As the sessions progressed, the children extended the time they stood still. When new records were set, they celebrated their accomplishments - exuding cheers and high fives. As the program drew to a close, these young, restless boys were capable of successfully standing virtually motionless and remaining silent for five minutes. Afterward, parents described improvements in their children that they attributed to the program. Frequently noted was greater self-control. One mother commented, "I feel my son now stops and focuses on what he is trying to accomplish. It's as if he doesn't jump right into things blindly anymore." Another parent remarked that her son had "learned to breathe, relax, and take control of himself." Individuals, including children, want to feel in control. An older graduate student I saw as a private client practiced self-control by eating one piece of popcorn at a time. As therapy progressed in lieu of racing his car down the road when angry, he claimed he would perform tai chi movements until he calmed down. Once practiced, strategies that promote self-control appear to be sustainable and were generalized to different settings outside of the program. For example, a mother notified me two years after her son had participated in the program that she had been contacted by his guidance counselor. The counselor relayed to the mother that her son had been making remarkable progress. The guidance counselor added that she asked the boy why he was doing so much better. The boy replied, "Miss Cheryl taught me how to control myself."

Leaders experience fewer stressors. An individual's position in a social hierarchy impacts their stress level. Children with autism are perceived as weak and easy targets for bullying. Contrary to an earlier animal study that coined the term "executive stress syndrome," it has been determined that humans who hold leadership positions experience less stress. Lower cortisol levels and lower levels of self-reported anxiety were found in government and military leaders than in those they supervised (Sherman et al., 2012). Dr. Sapolsky vividly provides evidence of this in his previously referenced documentary. Counselors can train children with autism in specific leadership skills and coordinate efforts with home and school to provide leadership opportunities. Parents and classroom teachers can guide and encourage children while they perform as leaders.

Building leadership skills empowers individuals to exercise more control. The program I developed was orchestrated to foster leadership. Leadership opportunities for those with autism should occur routinely throughout their day. An example would be allowing children to distribute snacks to younger children. Classroom duties and being in charge of animals could also be helpful. Responsibilities can increase as leadership skills develop. It is essential that the child be successful. Leadership responsibilities that the individual enjoys should not be removed as a disciplinary tactic. However tempting, it is likely counterproductive to take away or threaten to take away a leadership role that a child enjoys, for example, for not completing homework. The homework should be addressed as a separate issue. All of the children in the program were wiling to serve as leaders. The role was modified based on the child's age and demonstrated ability to assure success. At the end of the program, I received feedback from teachers that participants become more likely to raise their hand and volunteer in the classroom.

As direct services, psychological counseling would assist in training a child in self-control and leadership. The counselor can foster opportunities at school and in the home. Both will be beneficial in assisting the child to better regulate stress.

Chapter 17
MINIMIZING STRESSORS

A critical part of treatment is minimizing stressors. The frequency, intensity, and duration of psychosocial and physical stressors experienced by those with autism need to decrease. This can be accomplished by avoiding stressors or changing the stressful environment. Whenever conceivable, behavioral strategies should be created and implemented by the child with guidance and support from professional staff and parents. Regardless of its benefits, however, professionals and parents may be reluctant to relinquish control. Throughout my career I have repeatedly witnessed the dismal failures of professionally crafted behavioral plans. Some plans worked for a short time before collapsing; others never got off the ground. Occasionally, success was found in one setting, but not generalized to another. I can personally testify to the struggles one can face when trying to modify behavior. I acquired an adorable eight-week-old puppy. For training purposes, the animal had virtually all my attention in one room for most of nine days -rather ideal conditions. The pup outwitted, outlasted, and humbled me. I believe the major flaw was competing goals. The dog wanted her freedom, I wanted her contained. She chose to bark, I enjoyed silence. She urinated at will, I wanted unsoiled floors. Puppies, like children (and adults), have resources to get their way. The puppy yelped a piercing coyote-like howl when I left her unattended. Her crying, like that of an infant or child, was painfully loud and distressing. It lasted forever. Crying and temper tantrums have a purpose and can be difficult to bear. It is understandable why parents (and trainers like myself) give up and give in. As another resource, when resisting change, animals and people can be cunning. For example, when something would momentarily distract me, like pouring a cup of coffee, the puppy would quietly slip away-vaporize. When I noted her absence, I would frantically dart about the house knowing she was likely going to engage in an undesirable behavior. More often than not, I was too late.

I have found for the most part, people are content with their behaviors-set in their ways. Those attempting to change another's behavior will likely be met with resistance and disappointment. It is not easy to change someone else's behavior, and children are no exception. If children are given ownership and control, they are less likely to rebel and behave appropriately. They need to be directed in methods to control the stressors in their environments.

That being said, overall, it may be better to try to change the environment rather than the person. Manipulating the antecedents that evoke the stress response will likely be easier, quicker, and more effective. Critics argue, however, that when working with children, making adaptations pampers and mollycoddles them, resulting in their being ill-prepared for the real world. They claim children have to learn to "deal with it". Unfortunately, due to a malfunctioning stress response, without treatment and training, those with autism can't and won't.

In attempting to change the environment, accurately identifying the individual's stressors is an important first step. Some are obvious, others not. Stressors for those with autism, as previously detailed, can be markedly different from others. When working with children, the efforts of a multidisciplinary team including the parent(s) and child, when appropriate, increase the likelihood of correctly identifying stressors. Input from psychologists, counselors, behavioral therapists, occupational therapists, and teachers should be solicited and can provide critical information in the identification process.

Both sensory and social stressors need to be identified and addressed. Recent technology can be incredibly important in the identification of sensory and social stressors. A Virtual Environment (VE) designed to measure sensory reactions to visual, auditory, and olfactory input can provide objective data regarding sensory impairments. It can also determine reactions to social stressors. The reactions to the stimuli have effectively been used to differentiate those with autism from those who do not (Alcañiz et al., 2020). This invaluable tool can also serve to measure an individual's response to treatment.

Once identified, stressors need to be addressed. Behavioral interventions that focus on modifying sensory stimuli and social skills training that focuses directly on stress-generating interactions can provide significant relief. Counselor, occupational therapist, and behavioral specialist working closely with teachers and parents could be very beneficial in minimizing stressors. Those with autism are stressed by overloads of auditory, visual, and tactile stimuli. They can be trained to better identify stressors in their environments. They can be taught different methods of modifying the stressors or ways to avoid them. The following provides examples of modifying sensory stimuli including sound, light, and touch in the environment.

Auditory. There is a growing awareness of the benefits of quiet surroundings. I recently observed a sign in a hospital hallway that read, "Quiet hallways promote rest and healing. Shhhhh! Quiet please." Turning down loud car speakers or turning off the blare of a television can immediately restore tranquility and relieve stress. Caretakers can monitor the noise of environments within which children with autism are navigating. In extremely noisy places like school cafeterias, the stress of the environment can be overwhelming. Plans to address noisy surroundings should be in place. Headsets, which have become more fashionable, may be used to protect ears and reduce noise. Individuals should be given the choice, whenever possible, in whether they choose to wear them.

Visual. Light can be stressful. When driving east toward the rising sun, the glare can be blinding. You may lose sight of oncoming vehicles and your place on the road. Imagine that sensation occurring periodically throughout your day. At a conference I attended, the keynote speaker with autism wore a baseball cap while addressing us from the podium. He explained to the audience that the cap shielded his eyes from the overhead lights. Fluorescent lighting in classrooms and offices can produce an uncomfortable glare and can be replaced with tubes of incandescent lighting. Darker shades on table lamps and on windows can also provide relief. Additionally, dimmers on light switches, sunglasses, and hats can instantly and safely relieve the stress caused by bright, glaring light.

Tactile. Tactile sensitivity, as previously addressed, is a particular area of concern for those with autism. Certain textiles like wool can be rough and irritating. Clothing tags scratch sensitive skin and manufacturers are eliminating them. Anything that scratches or otherwise irritates the skin can cause discomfort. It is emphasized that the sensations are amplified and enduring in those with autism. Within reason, these children should be allowed to dress comfortably.

Behavioral and occupational therapists are key personnel in cooperatively devising and executing a plan to address sensory stimuli. Noise, light, and touch can be better controlled in home and school settings. Quiet surroundings, proper lighting, and comfortable clothing can minimize stressors.

In treating autism it is essential that their environments become less stressful. It is acknowledged that even with a concerted effort to minimize stressors, they will invariably occur. It would be beneficial, however, if there were fewer. When we are unable to provide relief, we want to reduce the damage. Coping with unavoidable stressors can be addressed by promoting relaxation.

Chapter 18
PROMOTING RELAXATION

Relaxation is a necessity, not a luxury -not an indulgence. Training individuals in methods of relaxation is the second prong of my model. Those with autism will benefit from being taught how to relax. This, however, can be a monumental feat since even those without autism can have problems relaxing, and I am no exception. Sitting quietly is not my nature. In elementary school my report card read "wiggles and talks too much." I dreaded the directive to rest after recess. I would reluctantly position my head on my outstretched arm which was draped on my desk for what seemed an eternity. Time was devoted to relaxing and doing nothing. In today's classroom, this would be considered a waste of time. The relaxation response tempers biological reactions to stressors and restores balance to our systems (allostasis) after stressful occurrences. An individual's system can be better trained to do so. There is more than one way to promote relaxation.

Empirical research identifies a variety of meditative practices that are effective in regulating stress. Meditative exercises such as tai chi, qigong (a more stationary form of tai chi), and yoga promote relaxation and can be practiced by those with autism. A combination of approaches has been shown to be more effective than any single approach (Tang et al., 2007). Modifications will need to be made dependent upon the individual's age, circumstances, and functioning levels. Critical factors like pregnancy and the fragile nature of infants will also need to be carefully considered and are addressed next.

Chapter 19
TREATING STRESS DURING PREGNANCY

Prenatal stress can impact the developing fetus and later interfere with the newborn's ability to regulate stress. Ideally, women would address high stress hormone levels before becoming pregnant. Once pregnant, the fetus is affected by the mother's stress hormones, and excessively high stress hormone levels need to be lowered. In particular, three populations of pregnant women who are at greater risk of having a baby, who will later be diagnosed with autism, would be advised to seek treatment:

- women who already have a child with autism (Buss et al., 2010),
- women with closely spaced pregnancies (Cheslack-Postava et al., 2011),
- women with abnormal cortisol levels during pregnancy (Ram et al., 2018).

Not only do these three groups of women share a higher risk of giving birth to a child with autism, but they also share another common denominator: the women are all more likely to have abnormally high stress hormone levels. The first two groups are caretakers, which makes them particularly vulnerable to stress (Epel et al., 2004). The third group is composed of women with abnormal levels of stress hormones who gave birth to fetuses who were later more likely to be diagnosed with autism. In one of the studies in this group, maternal plasma cortisol was measured at 15, 19, 25, 31, and 37 weeks' gestation in 84 pregnant women. ASD symptoms were assessed in their 5-year-old children. Fetal exposure to abnormal levels of maternal cortisol was associated with higher levels of ASD symptoms found in males only (Ram et al., 2018). In a study of 2900 pregnant women with high levels of maternal stress during pregnancy, stressful events during pregnancy significantly predicted autistic traits in the offspring at age two. Once again, this was found in males only (Ronald et al., 2011).

Women who are pregnant or considering becoming pregnant need to be aware of the potential consequences of stress on a developing fetus. Only a few generations ago, cigarette smoking was not a recognized health risk. Pregnant women smoked without hesitation. They now know that smoking endangers the well-being of their developing fetus and can make an informed chose. Like information about the dangers of smoking, information regarding stress and pregnancy needs to be widely disseminated. Women with high stress levels, whether due to life styles or genes, should be encouraged by their physicians to seek treatment. More support is needed by the family and community. Treatment should be affordable and widely available. As previously cautioned, consultation with a physician is recommended before beginning any program or following any advice of this author. The reader is reminded that treatment is not for the purpose of curing or preventing autism, but for mitigating and preventing symptoms that are caused or exacerbated by stress. Evidence indicates that when a mother relaxes, the effects on the fetus are immediate. While practicing a relaxation technique, pregnant women demonstrated reductions in psychological stress as measured by heart rate, skin conductance, and cortisol levels. The relaxation of the mother triggered significant alterations in fetal cardiac patterns and affected other fetal neurobehavior (DiPietro et al., 2008).

Training a pregnant woman to better address stress empowers her. The woman can execute more control once she is trained in methods to minimize stressors and relax. Feeling in control is a powerful regulator of stress. Although practices that reduce stress can be virtually free and are widely available, few pregnant women participate in routine activities that promote relaxation. A survey of pregnant women indicated the most commonly employed techniques included yoga (7.3%) and meditation (4.5%), though few reported using relaxation techniques daily (2.7%) (DiPietro et al., 2008). Exercise can also reduce stress but is not a substitute for a routine of meditative practices. Individuals who meditated regularly, although they were heavier and exercised less, were more relaxed and had longer telomeres than peers who exercised more frequently (Alda et al., 2016).

Pregnant women are part of a community and social support indeed helps buffer stress (Heinrichs et al., 2003). It takes a village to raise a child, but the village needs to rally prior to the child's birth. Family and friends can offer invaluable support to reduce the expectant mother's stress. My mother often recalled an incident of community support extended to her while pregnant. Our family annually made a trip to an amusement park. With five children under tow, my mother packed a picnic lunch, and we were off to spend the day thrill-riding. She recollects that we all reluctantly returned to the picnic grounds for dinner, where a table had been set with hotdogs and hamburgers sizzling on the grill. It was a steamy July day, and my mother who barely reached five feet tall was pregnant with triplets. A stranger at a nearby table approached her and offered a platter that held a juicy steak that he insisted was for her. Years later she would gently glow with a soft smile while recalling that gesture of kindness. An extra effort to nurture pregnant women can make a difference.

Employers, physicians, and mental health providers can also assist in reducing the stress of pregnant women. Obstetricians, in particular, can be instrumental in raising awareness and recommending treatment for stress. Stress levels need to be monitored throughout the pregnancy. Government and private agencies can promote programs to assist pregnant women, which would reduce medical claims and future educational expenses. Programs for pregnant women, like the Silver Sneakers program offered to senior citizens, could provide substantial savings to insurance companies. Indeed, it takes a village.

Chapter 20
TREATING INFANTS

Upon birth the primary focus for treating stress should shift from the mother to the newborn. Infants with a dysregulation of the HPA axis need to be identified and treated. Elevated stress levels can be detected in infants with safe, noninvasive measures. To more directly assess a neonate's stress levels, a battery of assessments should be administered along with the APGAR assessment (which assesses physical health). This stress protocol would provide a measure of mental health that complements the physical health assessment routinely conducted on newborns. Stress is a critical component of mental health of infants that needs to be conscientiously addressed.

Several stress-related biomarkers previously discussed can assist in the assessment process to determine those infants at greater risk for later being diagnosed with autism. Those identified with elevated stress levels should receive treatment immediately. The following indicators have been used in approved research studies to assess stress in infants:

- Abnormal cortisol levels taken from samples of an infant's saliva or hair can indicate a higher risk for later being diagnosed with autism. Newborn infants' hair cortisol levels reflect chronic maternal stress during the pregnancy (Romero-Gonzalez et al., 2018).
- An infant's cry can help differentiate infants who are at greater risk of later being diagnosed with autism. The distinguishable higher-than-

normal cry of these infants is more aversive to adults, and technology can reliably detect differences.

- Shorter-than-normal telomeres in infants can indicate a higher risk for autism. Shorter telomeres are markers for exposure to prenatal stress. Abnormal reactions of the pupil can assist in identifying infants who will later be diagnosed with autism.
- The failure to habituate can be detected in infants and is a distinctive characteristic of those with autism.

Infants depend on us for their very survival. They have virtually no control over their environment and no choice in the people who care for them. As with all of us they are exposed to daily stressors, but unlike us, they can do little or nothing about them. Infants born with high stress levels need treatment, and the earlier the better. Preterm infants are particularly at risk of high stress levels due to pain from needles, a noisy neonatal intensive care unit (NICU), and lack of holding. An infant vocalizes its discomfort through crying but cannot articulate the source of the discomfort. Caretakers find themselves involved in a guessing game trying to identify the stressors. To further obfuscate matters, as noted previously, crying does not always accompany stress. Without relief the stressor remains capable of altering brain neuroarchitecture and genes. DNA methylation of stress-related genes including NR3C1 is affected by the stress of pain exposure (Provenzi et al., 2015). These at-risk infants are particularly vulnerable to harm since this is a time of rapid brain growth.

In the quest to better regulate stress in infants, the same directives apply in the treatment model, minimize stressors and promote relaxation. There are, of course, distinct differences in how treatment is delivered. Both physical and psychological concerns of the infant need to be addressed. Psychologists and occupational therapists become key professional personnel. It has been determined that stress is a health concern that impairs cognitive flexibility as early as infancy (Seehagen et al., 2015). This cognitive impairment puts them "at-risk of developing a delay or special need that may affect their development or impede their education" (IDEA, Part C). Part C of IDEA provides for early intervention (EI) services - Child Find to assist at-risk children from birth to their third birthdays.

There is a paucity of research devoted specifically to treating stress in infants identified as having higher-than-normal stress levels. It has been established that infants who are born very preterm are significantly more likely to have altered HPA axis functioning at three, eight, and eighteen months, and at seven years (Grunau et al., 2007) Interventions are available to enhance the clinical course of premature infants. Treatment can also be beneficial with full-term infants who have higher-than-normal levels of stress hormones.

Minimizing Stressors. An infant's sensory systems can serve as pathways to regulate stress. This can occur with modifications to the environment at home and in other settings. Each infant's response to treatment may vary, which makes progress monitoring essential. What works for one may not work for another. Stimuli can be modified through a variety of channels, but focusing on decreasing auditory, visual, and tactile stimuli is recommended. Noises can be silenced; sounds can be deadened. Noisy neonatal units are a concern being addressed in many hospitals. As previously mentioned the stress response is active in infants. Their systems react to auditory stimuli adding to stressors. While traveling, infants and toddlers are strapped in car seats positioned near rear speakers. The driver can switch the music from the back to the front of the car. In the home, lowering the volume or turning off a stereo or television quickly reduces noise. Playing music from a harp was associated with lower cortisol levels in premature infants (Schwilling et al., 2015). Visual stimuli, particularly bright and direct lighting, can be stressful. Overhead lights positioned above a supine infant can be bright. There is evidence that premature infants make better progress when spending more time in prone positions (Candia et al., 2014). Although the factors that could account for this change were not identified, lighting may have contributed. Dimly lit floor and table lamps can protect an infant from the stress of harsh overhead lighting, particularly when the infant is lying on its back. When bright lighting is unavoidable, infants' eyes can be shielded with a hand or some other source of shade. An infant may find relief in a darkened room that simulates the womb. Research needs to be conducted to determine the consequences of lighting on infant stress.

Tactile stimuli are a primary source of stress for those with autism. Their reactions to touch are often extreme. Tactile sensations are also likely to evoke similar reactions in highly stressed at-risk infants. Diapers, clothing, bedding, and towels are all potential sources of irritation and discomfort. Something smooth like satin may be more soothing than cotton. Reactions to different fabrics on high-risk infants need to be investigated. Careful consideration is needed, since unlike older children, infants can't refuse to get dressed.

Promoting Relaxation. Infants need to relax. Since meditating is not a viable option, different methods for assisting highly stressed infants are needed. Infants at high-risk for being diagnosed with autism can be targeted as infants. For most of us, being held and gently touched promotes relaxation (Feldman et al., 2010). According to the literature, this holds true for infants. A review was conducted of eight randomized-controlled studies that assessed the impact of massage on vagal activity of preterm infants. There was an increase in vagal tone in all trials, indicating involvement of the parasympathetic system which promotes relaxation (Niemi, 2017). Preterm infants receiving massage therapy showed fewer stress behaviors and less agitation from the first day of the massage until the fifth and final day of the experiment (Hernandez-Reif et al., 2007). In a review of 19 studies of distressed infants who cried excessively, massage was determined to be beneficial (Carnes et al., 2018). Infants with a medical condition, gastroesophageal reflux disease (GERD), showed decreases in cortisol levels with massage therapy. GERD occurs when the muscle that connects the esophagus to the stomach does not operate properly. Infants with GERD, who did not have massage therapy, had increases in cortisol levels over time (Neu et al., 2013).

Although the majority of research documents improvements from infant massage, there are studies that indicate massage can elevate stress hormone levels. A study was conducted to explore the effect of administering massage with and without other sensory stimulation on full-term infants. In the massage-only group, eye contact or vocalizations with the infant were prohibited. It was determined that when massage is administered with only tactile stimulation, stress hormone levels increase. In the other group, when massage was administered normally, stress hormone levels decreased (White-Traut et al., 2009). In viewing these outcomes, the lack of eye contact may have been a confounding variable that actually contributed to the rise in stress hormones. It may be mistaken to assume that the massage was responsible for the rise in stress hormones, in whole or in part. A compelling video entitled the Still-Face Experiment, conducted at Harvard University by Dr. Edward Tronick, depicts the highly stressful reactions of infants who do not get feedback from the faces of their mothers. The infants become visibly distressed when their mothers ignore their attempts to communicate. Typically, when massage is administered, there would be social interaction which makes this issue of less concern.

Since tactile sensitivity and social interaction can be stressful for those with autism, the reactions to massage with infants at high risk for autism are difficult to predict. Physiological and behavioral reactions would need to be closely monitored. As previously noted, infants do not always cry when stressed, and the infants' behavioral reactions did not differ when stressed during massage. Careful monitoring with instruments that will detect the onset of stressful reactions is needed, and frequent measurements of cortisol levels should also be taken. If an infant were to react negatively, the intervention should cease. Infants at higher risk for autism may not habituate, and desensitization therapies could render further harm.

Massage therapy has been successfully adapted with positive outcomes for children with autism. Social and sensory issues can improve (Silva et al.,

2015). With adaptations the impact of massage on infants, who are at higher risk for later being diagnosed with autism, would likely be even greater due to earlier intervention. One set of guidelines for infant massage is provided online by the Mayo Clinic.

Another intervention for treating stress in infants is known as skin-to-skin contact (SSC) or "kangaroo care," whereby the newborn is immediately placed on the mother's chest. Infants randomized to SSC had a significantly lower salivary cortisol reactivity at one month (p=0.01) (Mörelius et al., 2015). Remarkably, SSC shows long-term effects on stress resilience that have been documented through age 10 (Feldman et al., 2014). Research is needed on the impact of SSC on newborns at higher risk for autism. SSC as standard protocol for these infants could reap substantial benefits.

Consistent with these findings, physical closeness of the mother while in the hospital impacts infant stress levels. When mother and baby remain in the same hospital room throughout their stay, the infants with constant contact have lower salivary cortisol levels than those who are with their mothers part-time (De Bernardo et al., 2018). In another study, auditory stimulation using a maternal heartbeat was found to reduce cortisol after a needle prick (Kurihara et al., 1996). The artificial heartbeat could perhaps prevent stressful reactions when mother is absent.

Swaddled bathing is another promising intervention for treating highly stressed infants. When being bathed the infant is loosely wrapped in cloth to help maintain body temperature and reduce stress. Behavioral stress symptoms are observed less frequently in infants who are wrapped when being bathed (Çaka & Gözen, 2017).

For infants with abnormal stress levels, the findings regarding treatment are promising. Multimodal approaches to reducing stress are recommended. The research indicates excessive stress in infants can be accurately identified, closely monitored, and (with caution) successfully treated. Early intervention can impact stress in childhood.

Chapter 21
TREATING STRESS IN CHILDREN

The current available research suggests meditative practices, massage therapy, and pet therapy would categorically be suitable and beneficial for children with autism. Preliminary findings indicate that symptoms of those with autism can be curtailed, and children with autism can be trained in methods to relax.

Meditative Practices. Meditation alters brain activity. When meditating, the amygdala reacts less to obtrusive auditory stimuli (Brefczynskik-Lewis et al., 2007). Although a variety of meditative practices can promote relaxation in the general population, the techniques need to be modified to accommodate those with autism. If early intervention is to succeed, interventions need to be adapted for children with high activity levels and short attention spans. My feasibility studies showed tai chi could be successfully adapted. Accommodations were made and because the children were upright with face-to-face contact, a social element was in place. This is important for children with autism. Unexpectedly, a team spirit emerged and as they strutted down the hallways they touted that they were members of the "Tai Chi Team". This is an advantage of this form of meditative practice. Another advantage of tai chi is that it allows for children to move throughout most of the session. The group typically moved in unison, similar to a marching band, but very slowly. The slow-moving exercises were interchanged with more physically vigorous activity to avoid restlessness. Empirical research to assess the impact of tai chi on children with autism is needed and feasible since it has been demonstrated that the practice can be adapted for use with this population.

Yoga. Yoga can also be practiced by those with autism and is appropriate for children. It has grown in popularity and is now being offered in many elementary and secondary schools. A study shows that after an eight-week yoga program, sensory impairments and other symptoms significantly improve for children with autism (Sotoodeh, 2017).

Mindfulness-based stress reduction (MBSR). MBSR is a meditative exercise that focuses on remaining in the present and not being judgmental. Meditative exercises focus on the breath. Exhaling in any program is the key to relaxation. Improved sensory processing and a more consistent attentional focus were evident in the general population after eight weeks of mindfulness meditation (Kilpatrick et al., 2011; Ridderinkhof et al., 2018). MBSR when practiced by parents of children with autism had positive outcomes for both parties. Among the outcomes, the parents were less stressed and depressed; the children showed improvements in attention (Neece, C. 2013).

Massage Therapy. Counter to expectations massage therapy has been found to be very effective in reducing stress. As previously mentioned, tactile sensitivity is the most prevalent sensory abnormality in those with autism with rates that have been estimated to be over 95% (Silva & Schalock, 2013a). Massage therapy, however, has been shown to decrease stress, resulting in lower cortisol, decreased anxiety, and lower systolic/diastolic blood pressure (Pinar & Afsar, 2015; Field, 2014). In a randomized controlled study of the effects of massage on children with autism, 103 preschool children were treated with therapeutic massage for five months. The massage was applied daily by parents and weekly by therapists. The parents were trained and supervised by the therapists. Results of the intervention indicated a reduction in tactile abnormalities and improved social skills, language, and behavior. Assessment indicated that at five months: tactile abnormalities were reduced by approximately 50%; autism severity was reduced by 16%; and 6% of the children no longer met the criteria for having autism (Silva & Schalock, 2013b). The study was successfully replicated and yielded similar results (Silva et al., 2015). Longer-term treatment was even more promising. Mean autism severity continued to decrease, tactile responses were less intense, and at 24 months 26% of the children were reported to have "moved out of the autistic range" (Silva, 2016). Even though those with autism may initially be averse to touch, a therapeutic massage program has been developed that successfully improves symptoms of autism.

Pet Therapy. Children with autism are plagued by chronic anxiety and normally experience more stress during social interactions than typical children. Regardless of their inept social skills, they still want friends. A vehicle that promotes relaxation for these children while they socialize has been identified. Social anxiety is significantly reduced in children with autism when they are accompanied by an animal. As mentioned previously, skin conductance response (SCR), a measure of physiological arousal, was determined to be significantly higher in those with autism under a variety of social conditions (O'Haire et al., 2015). The presence of companion animals in a social context reduced autonomic arousal. Unlike their TD peers, they showed a 43% reduction in SCRs during free play when animals were included. Parents and teachers reported global improvements in social skills for children with autism when animals were kept in the school classroom (O'Haire et al., 2014; O'Haire et al., 2015). Stuffed animals may serve as a viable alternative where live pets are prohibited. Further research is needed to assess their potential viability.

Meditative practices, massage therapy, and pet therapy are safe and effective methods that promote relaxation and can be used with children who have autism. These interventions can be complemented with other methods of relaxation like hobbies. The impact exercise has on cortisol levels varies dependent upon the exercise intervention (Wegner et al., 2019). Hobbies in-

cluding arts and crafts, music, and drama are encouraged. Unstructured social interactions can be relaxing. As a part of my program, the children played
with Legos while awaiting for others to arrive. Engagement in extracurricular
activities should be initiated judiciously since structured play can be a potent
source of stress for children with autism. Keeping social activities simple
with few rules is recommended. Free play is less stressful (Corbett et al.,
2009). Group activities like scouting, swimming, fishing, and hiking typically have fewer rules and are less competitive than team sports. They may
be better suited for children with autism since, generally speaking, more
rules equal more stress for them. Competitive sports like Little League Baseball have many rules. To further aggravate matters, gross motor coordination
is impaired in approximately 20% of children with ASD. These physically
awkward children also have more difficulty with social relationships
than other children with ASD (Pusponegoro et al., 2016). Their lack of
athleticism can be a detriment to a team's success, setting the child up
as a target to be bullied.

Regardless of the methodology, promoting relaxation for children with
autism is beneficial. It is advantageous to know that unlike the risks associated with pharmaceuticals, these interventions are considered to be safe. Relaxation should be encouraged beginning in infancy and be continued
throughout the life span. Additional precautions and adaptations are
necessary for pregnant women and infants; monitoring by a physician
is considered essential.

Chapter 22
PARENTS' STRESS

Stress is contagious — the stress response is activated in 40% of the people who are observing the stress of someone else close to them. While we are observing the stress of another person, our cortisol levels increase significantly (Engert et al., 2014). For children with autism, this can mean double jeopardy. If they evoke stress in others, they are likely to be recipients of more stress in return. The stress of caregivers, therefore, is influential in the well-being of a child with autism.

Addressing the stress of parents, however, is a monumental task that, for the most part, extends beyond the scope of this book. Since parents' stress does impact their children, I am providing a brief overview of the reasons for concern and treatment guidelines.

The excessive stress of caregivers is well-documented in the literature. As a reviewer for the Journal of Autism and Developmental Disorders, I am far more frequently asked to evaluate submissions on parents' stress than submissions on their children's. All parenting is stressful, but raising a child with autism can evoke an inordinate amount of stress. Mothers of children with autism report significantly greater levels of psychological stress than mothers of typically developing (TD) children or of those with other types of disabilities (Abbeduto et al., 2004; Hayes et al., 2013). Their stress is not without consequences. It is firmly established that stress is associated with an increased risk of cardiovascular disease and heart disease is the leading cause of death for women in the United States (Yusuf, 2004). According to the Centers for Disease Control and Prevention (CDC), heart disease is responsible for the deaths of about one in every four females. Approximately two-thirds of those who die suddenly, had no prior symptoms. Chronically stressed mothers of children with autism exhibit alterations in immune and cholesterol biomarkers that reflect increased cardiovascular risk (Aschbacher et al., 2017). This configuration does not bode well for mothers of children with autism.

Stress impacts our health by modulating the rate of cellular aging. Not only does stress damage caregivers' cardiovascular systems, but research indicates it also shortens their telomeres. As noted earlier, telomeres are protective caps at the ends of DNA that shorten with age. Mothers of children with autism are highly stressed and have shorter-than-normal telomeres (Nelson et al., 2015). Mothers who care for chronically ill children also have significantly higher levels of stress and shorter telomeres. The women with the highest levels of stress have telomeres shorter on average by the equivalent of at least one decade of additional aging. The more years of caregiving, the shorter the mother's telomere length (Epel et al., 2004). Stress presents a very real threat for these women.

Treatment. It should be better known that parents, as well as their children with autism, are entitled to "counseling and training" as a related service under federal law (Section 300.34 of IDEA). When providing services, counselors can apply the same treatment model for adults as previously described for children. Individual and group counseling would be conducted within the same framework-minimize stressors and promote relaxation. I have successfully applied this model in both individual and group settings with women as well as children. The adult programs clinically address psychosocial stressors, use meditative techniques for relaxation, and incorporate therapeutic massage. In past programs each of these treatment components was delivered within one hourly session. The participants attended regularly and provided me with positive feedback; they repeatedly noted that they had experienced reduced stress.

Additionally, parents can participate in community programs and recreational activities that promote relaxation. This is particularly important if the mothers of children with autism are pregnant or planning to become pregnant. As a general practice, obstetricians should routinely monitor cortisol levels in pregnant women. Offerings like yoga, tai chi, and massage therapy should be made readily available. A large randomized trial program was conducted using a meditative technique, Mindfulness-Based Stress Reduction (MBSR), to relax mothers of children with autism. Results indicate: significant reductions in stress, improved sleep, and better satisfaction with life. The effect sizes were medium to large for depression and anxiety from baseline to the 6-month follow-up. Interestingly, similar to the massage therapy, the MBSR intervention was also provided by parents who were trained and supervised by mental health professionals (Dykens et al., 2014).

Stress regulation programs that would offer services for adults and children separately, but simultaneously, could exponentially reap greater benefits. As previously discussed, telomere length is an indicator of wellness and longevity that is impacted by stress. In the research on telomeres, the only group of children with autism whose telomeres were normal had been in a family counseling program (Li et al., 2014).

Parents of children who participated in my second feasibility study were asked to remain during their child's training. The parents gathered in a separate room while waiting. They repeatedly claimed that being with others who shared similar problems was helpful. Among the parents and children a camaraderie emerged that extended into the community. As previously mentioned, while waiting, the parents socialized and invited each other's children to their homes for "play dates."

These programs can be spearheaded in the community by local advocacy groups and backed by national organizations like Autism Speaks. The services can be held in local YMCAs, schools, and churches and coordinated with mental health agencies. The benefits would also likely be cost effective to insurance companies and taxpayers. There are no easy fixes, but the stress of parenting children with autism needs to be relieved. As flight attendants advise on aircraft, parents should put their oxygen masks on first before assisting others.

Chapter 23
ASSESSMENT & DIAGNOSIS

The body's reactions to stressors can be detected and measured. Tools are currently available that can determine stress levels prior to birth. Stress that an infant was exposed to during pregnancy can be detected from a hair sample. Although not yet used routinely for examination purposes, there are instruments that have been approved by numerous reputable ethics committees for research. Childhood stress is now recognized as a health concern, and these instruments can accurately identify the problem in both medical and educational settings. Data collection regarding the dysregulation of HPA axis functioning, critical for the regulation of stress, should become a part of routine examinations in child care. Obstetricians, pediatricians, and family physicians can screen large numbers of children accurately, efficiently, and economically for stress-related concerns. Methods are currently available to screen high-risk infants for elevated stress levels. Methods of detection that would be practical for pediatrician and family physician use with children in the general population include assessment of cortisol levels, telomere length, electrodermal activity (EDA), and heart rate variability. Cortisol levels can be determined from saliva or hair samples (McEwen et al., 2019). Exposure to chronic stress is associated with shorter telomere length in genes which can be sampled using several different non-invasive measures (Lai et al., 2018; Montpetitie et al., 2014; Révész D. et al., 2014). Pediatricians or family physicians can be instrumental in detecting stress levels. Physicians can non-invasively determine if biomarkers are present indicating elevated stress levels. If higher stress levels are indicated, a child can be referred to the special education office of the local school district to determine the need for services. A multi-disciplinary team would recommend the appropriate assessments. A psychological assessment would routinely be a part of the assessment battery. Once services are instituted, physicians can then assist in monitoring the effects of treatment on stress hormone levels. Additionally, doctors would treat stress-related health concerns like irritable bowel syndrome (IBS). An overview of the intervention process for identification and treatment could proceed as follows:

As part of a child's routine examination, the pediatrician screens stress hormone levels. A child with stress indices that are abnormal is then referred by the parent(s) to the local school district.

The school then convenes a child study team to proceed with further evaluation of the child to make treatment and placement decisions. Since stress adversely impacts brain functioning, academic performance, and social/emotional well-being, a comprehensive evaluation including a psychological assessment, when appropriate, should be conducted (Ljung et al., 2009). A comprehensive evaluation would include assessments of cognition, sensory regulation, social interactions, emotional adjustment, executive functioning and academic performance.

A wide range of uncharacteristic symptoms that can be caused or exacerbated by stress, particularly in those with autism, have been overlooked and will likely remain undetected with current assessment tools. Traditional psychometric instruments to determine stress levels may be inadequate. There are a number of reasons these assessments need to be revised. Additionally, behavioral symptoms of stress may or may not manifest. Some children suffer from stressors in silence, conforming in social situations so as not to draw attention. When interviewing, parents may be hesitant to disclose stressful events that are occurring in the home. Another problem in current methods of assessment, may be the expertise and subjectivity of the examiner while conducting interviews. All of these factors can influence the results of the evaluation. The Stress Survey Schedule for Persons with Autism and Other Developmental Disorders is an instrument developed to assess eight dimensions of stress in those with autism. This instrument could assist in determining specific stressors that need to be targeted. A best practices model for assessment purposes needs to be developed.

Remarkably, new technology has developed an instrument that can recreate a person's biological reaction to sensory stimulation and social interactions in a virtual environment. The reaction is then measured by assessing changes in electrodermal activity (EDA). The reactions could differentiate between those with autism and those who did not have autism. These findings provide objective, physical evidence of greater autonomic arousal to sensory stimuli in children with autism. Due to greater control afforded by this instrument, the ability to obtain valid data from EDA is substantially increased over previous findings (Raya et al., 2020). This quantitative measure can become incredibly useful as a diagnostic tool and in monitoring progress.

Once the evaluation is completed, the team determines if a child is eligible for special education services. A dual diagnoses, e.g. Autism and Other Health Impaired may best describe the condition. After diagnosis, an Individual Education Plan (IEP) would be developed to address the child's needs. Those children with extreme stress and functional impairments who do not have autism may meet IDEA eligibility criteria solely under the category of Other Health Impaired. Those who are not eligible for special education services may be served with an accommodation plan under federal statute, Section 504 of the Rehabilitation Act of 1973.

Mental health services to address stress should be included in all treatment plans. The pediatrician can assist in monitoring progress of stress levels. Plans include interventions to target specific stressors, strategies to prevent or minimize future stressors, and training in relaxation.

For identification purposes I propose a distinct category for classifying stress which I suggest be called - "Chronic Stress Disorder" (CSD). A chronic stress disorder would be defined as a condition in which elevated levels of stress hormones are detected for six months or longer. The disorder is due to a dysregulation of the HPA axis or exposure to extreme stress. The disorder contributes to impairments in cognition, social/emotional functioning, and sensory regulation, all of which can impact educational performance.

Due to the unusual nature of stress in individuals with autism, caution should be exercised so that their stress does not continue to be underestimated. This book can and should provide guidance and assistance to help prevent that from occurring. Organizations like Autism Speaks can oversee and help ensure that the identification and treatment procedures are suitable and effective for children with autism.

Chapter 24
PREVENTING STRESS GLOBALLY

Stress should not continue to be passed blindly from one generation to the next. The stress transmitted through our life styles and our genes predisposes our offspring to lives overwrought with stress. The American Psychological Association reports stress has increased annually throughout the past decade; those with autism, in particular, are paying a price. A nationwide campaign to protect future generations is needed. This vicious cycle can be broken in one generation.

Fortunately, there appears to be a raised consciousness within our society regarding stress. People are trying to relax. Mainstream America no longer considers yoga as voodoo practiced by old hippies. We would be sadly mistaken, however, if we thought rushing to the YMCA for a one-hour Monday night yoga class is going to fix matters. I once attended a crowded yoga class where exercises were accompanied by hip-hop music. Yoga does have benefits particularly regarding stress and can serve as one of many tools in the toolbox. Babies born with autism who undergo less stress during child rearing are likely to have fewer and less debilitating symptoms. The methods previously proposed targeted individuals or small groups with autism. Similar methods can be extended to help prevent stress in the general population. Less stress in the world would positively influence those with autism directly and indirectly, immediately, and in the future.

Prevention During Infancy. All newborns should be routinely examined to detect abnormal stress levels with a battery similar to the APGAR. Cortisol levels, telomere length, pupillary eye reflex, and the pitch of their cries can all assist in detecting the problem. After birth, stress hormones that the infant was exposed to in utero can be detected by the cortisol levels found in a hair sample. These diagnostic procedures are non-invasive and have been used safely. Any infant with an indicator of abnormal stress hormone levels should receive immediate attention as detailed in Chapter 18. A brief overview follows. Humans, beginning at birth, are wired to react and stop reacting to stressors. For all newborns, quiet, subdued settings with natural light can help prevent stimulus overload. Bright lights and clamoring machines should only be in operation when essential. With nurturing, we can offset the barrage of stressors faced by newborns. Having mothers remain in close proximity to their newborns helps prevent stress. Holding an infant restores calmness (Feldman et al., 2010). The extended family that assisted with willing arms may not be available, but supervised volunteers or paid staff can serve as surrogates to cuddle babies. This practice is occurring in some hospital settings and can be extended to the community.

Another positive practice that serves infants has begun: parents are now more likely to work from home. For those who can't remain at home, employers are inviting babies to the workplace. These practices will reduce infant stress in the general population.

Prevention During Early Childhood. When infants or toddlers transition from their homes to outside settings away from their parent's direct care, the child can become stressed. Larger, community child care centers have been found to be more stressful than home daycare settings (Gunnar et al., 2010). I chose a home daycare setting when initially returning to work and later transitioned my daughter to a larger child care center. Prior to her move from a home daycare to a child care center, I visited several potential settings. For the most part, I found the centers noisy and overcrowded. There was a great deal of clamor and crying. I visited centers that were so overpopulated they looked like ant farms. I also observed social aggression that went unchecked. Although toddlers are often perceived as cute and cuddly, they are also aggressive. A movie entitled, "Babies", has no words, but vividly captures the nature of social interactions among toddlers. Toddlers bite, and they bite a lot. In my search I located one center that checked several of my boxes-it was clean, well-supervised, and near my workplace. During my second visit I asked a staff member what occurred when a child misbehaved. I was informed that the lights were turned out and the child was reprimanded for doing "the devil's work."

Eventually, I found a child care center that was owned and operated by a registered nurse and an administrator with a master's degree in early childhood education. Both interacted with the children throughout the day. The center employed a large, well-trained, and dedicated staff. The place was busy but not chaotic. It appeared stimulating but not overwhelming. Upset children were comforted without hesitation. The children followed a curriculum that changed activities every fifteen minutes. They were introduced to foreign languages, danced to live music, created art projects, and spent time frolicking outdoors. Although as a psychologist I initially had reservations regarding the highly structured environment, I concluded after three years of observation that children who are actively engaged play cooperatively and rarely show signs of distress. Attendance fees were reasonable, and the business operated successfully for decades.

The federal government issues child care licensing regulations. The regulations govern health and safety to protect children from illness and injury. Training in the areas of health and safety for child care providers is required. Twelve different topics are included in the training protocol, but none address mental health. The mental health of children also needs safeguarding. Physical and psychosocial stressors need to be addressed with the same vigilance as monkey bars and measles. Stress damages the brain.

It is important to differentiate what is causing stressful reactions in children who attend child care in centers rather than homes. Once the sources of additional stress are identified, then changes should be made. Sensory overload and social aggression are likely culprits. Environments need to change, and centers need adequate staff who are well-trained; staff members need to be better trained to execute interventions that prevent and relieve stressors. I recommend the following interventions.

Facilities can be made quieter and less chaotic in the following ways. Rooms can be constructed to better absorb sound. Fluorescent lighting should be replaced. Water play and other relaxing activities in designated quiet zones can be made available. Efforts to promote relaxation can become a part of daily routines. Short, frequent breaks that reduce both visual and auditory stimuli can calm children. I have observed preschoolers engage in a mindfulness intervention and was surprised at their willingness to cooperate for approximately twenty minutes. The children sat quietly and the room became noticeably calmer. There are a variety of mindfulness programs available for preschoolers.

Creating a closer connection with family as a routine part of each child's day would also likely lower stress. For example, family photos can be displayed in the classroom. Technology can also assist with videos of family members, and screen time can be shared. These interventions can be reassuring to children who are missing their family. Social interactions among the toddlers and preschoolers can be better monitored with lower adult to children ratios. In addition to serving infants, toddlers, and preschoolers determined to have excessive stress would likely be eligible for special education services through early intervention (EI) - Child Find. Parents can inquire about services through their local school district.

Prevention for School-Aged Children. There is a growing awareness that many youths experience levels of chronic stress so severe that their ability to succeed academically is undermined, their mental health functioning is compromised, and the likelihood of them engaging in behavior that puts their well-being at risk escalates (Hardy, 2003; Suldo et al., 2008; Conner et al., 2009). There are long-term consequences of toxic stress evident at birth that continue into childhood and endure throughout adulthood. In order to break that vicious cycle, children need to become less stressed.

The American Association of Pediatricians (AAP) is propelling a "seismic shift" in pediatric care due to revolutionary findings regarding childhood stress. The AAP now acknowledges that excessive stress is a health condition that changes brain structure and damages lifelong health. "I am so hopeful that looking at behavioral and emotional functioning and problems in kids will be a fundamental part of routine pediatric care-not extra, not less important than the physical exam, but an integral part of what it means to provide pediatric care," says AAP member Carol Cohen Weitzman, M.D., Director of Developmental Behavioral Pediatrics at Yale School of Medicine. The AAP represents 60,000 pediatricians who are undertaking a comprehensive initiative to identify, treat, and prevent toxic stress in children, and for good reason: stress is dangerous. Children from a variety of backgrounds commit suicide; a shared feature of those with suicidal ideations is an abnormal cortisol response (O'Connor et al., 2017). Among those individuals who reported a lifetime history of suicide attempts, over 70% had an anxiety disorder (Nepon et al., 2010). As mentioned previously, an estimated 40% of those with autism have anxiety disorders (van Steensel et al., 2011). As one might therefore predict, those with autism have higher suicide rates than normal (Hirvikoski et al., 2016.) It was recently determined that young people with autism were at over twice the risk of suicide than young people without autism (Kirby et al., 2019). The potential sources of stress for children include bullies who target and traumatize them in cyberspace and on school buses. As previously noted, children with autism are at a far greater risk of being bullied than others; they need to be better protected.

Federal, state, and local agencies can assist in preventing and treating the harm caused by stress in children. The AAP is spearheading a public health campaign to prevent and treat toxic stress in childhood. Both the United States Department of Education and the Centers for Disease Control and Prevention (CDC) currently have in operation programs to address the well-being of the nation's children. In order to coordinate the efforts of education leaders and health sectors, the CDC has initiated the Whole School, Whole Community, Whole Child (WSCC) model. The model, designed to align the common goals of both sectors, puts into action a whole-child approach to education. Efforts of the AAP to address toxic stress directly align with the goals of the WSCC initiative.

School systems are delegated to deliver health-related services to children, and for good reason. According to the CDC, "Schools have direct contact with more than 95% of our nation's young people aged 5-17 years, for about six hours per day and up to 13 critical years of their social, psychological, physical, and intellectual development." Government educational agencies can adapt health and physical education curriculums to address stress from the kindergarten through graduation. The school curriculum can become an effective vehicle for addressing stress. Information and guidance in minimizing stressors can be provided in health classes. Mindfulness exercises such as yoga, tai chi, and qigong for relaxation can be taught in physical education classes. A school-wide program can serve all children including those with special needs who require adaptive physical education. Trained school counselors and psychologists can serve as consultants and provide in-service programs for teachers, workshops for parents, and therapy for students. In a review of research on mindfulness-based interventions in schools, 11 of 13 studies reported positive improvements in well-being and fewer discipline problems (Martinez & Zhao, 2018; Zenner et al., 2014). Comprehensive programs to address stress can potentially assist an estimated 60 million students who attend school daily. Without assistance a significant percentage of these students will have extreme stress as an adult. With intervention, a substantial number can be helped and, in turn, produce healthier offspring. Community mental health providers can partner with school personnel and families. To individually and globally address stress, we need to minimize stressors and promote relaxation. My treatment model targets individuals with autism. My comprehensive plan can help prevent stress in the general population including those with autism. Revelatory information from neuroscientists and psychologists indicate the plan will work. Concisely, healthier children become healthier adults. Healthier adults will then give birth to healthier babies.

Unequivocal evidence documents that individuals with autism are experiencing an overload of stress that is damaging their brains and threatening their lives. This stress can and should be treated more effectively. A global effort can extend and improve the lives of those with autism beginning immediately. We can make a world of difference by *Taming Autism*.

REFERENCES

CHAPTER 14 - BENEFITS OF TREATMENT

Armanios, M., & Blackburn, E. H. (2012). The telomere syndromes. Nature Reviews. Genetics, 13(10), 693-704. doi:10.1038/nrg3246.

Asok, A., Bernard, K., Rosen, J., Dozier, M., & Roth, T., (2014). Infant caregiver experiences alter telomere length in the brain. PLOS ONE, e101437. doi:10.1371/journal.pone. 0101437.

Bhasin, M., Dusek, J., Chang, B., Joseph, M., Denninger, J.W., Fricchione, G.L., ...& Libermann, T.A., (2013). Relaxation response induces temporal transcriptome changes in energy metabolism, insulin secretion and inflammatory pathways. PLoS ONE, 8(5): e62817. doi:10.1371/journal.pone.0062817.

Blackburn, E. H. (2000). Telomere states and cell fates. Nature, 408(6808), 53-56.

Blackburn, E. H. (2010). Telomeres and telomerase: the means to the end (Nobel lecture). Angewandte Chemie, 49(41), 7405-7421,doi:10.1002/anie.201002387.

Bloss, E.B., Janssen, W..G., McEwen, B.S., & Morrison, J.H. (2010). Interactive effects of stress and aging on structural plasticity in the prefrontal cortex. The Journal of Neuroscience, 30(19), 6726-6731.

Daubenmier, J., Lin, J., Blackburn, E., Hecht, F. M., Kristeller, J., Maninger, N., ... Epel, E. (2012). Changes in stress, eating, and metabolic factors are related to changes in telomerase activity in a randomized mindfulness intervention pilot study. Psychoneuroendocrinology, 37(7), 917-928 doi:10.1016/j.psyneuen.2011.10.008.

Dusek, J., Otu, H., Wohlhueter, A., Bhasin, M., Zerbini, L.. Joseph, M., ... Liberman, T. (2008). Genomic counter-stress changes induced by the relaxation response. PLoS ONE, 3(7), e2576.

Esch, T., Fricchione, G. & Stefano, G. (2003). The therapeutic use of the relaxation response in stress-related diseases. Medical Science Monitor, 9, 23-34.

Hölzel, B.K., Carmody, J., Evans, K.C., Hoge, E.A., Dusek, J.A., Morgan, L., ... Lazar, S. (2010). Stress reduction correlates with structural changes in the amygdala. Social Cognitive and Affective Neuroscience, 5(1), 11-17.

Kim, S., Han, S., You, Y., Chen, D. J., & Campisi, J. (2003). The human telomere-associated protein TIN2 stimulates interactions between telomeric DNA tracts in vitro. EMBO Reports, 4(7), 685-691.

Kolb, B., and Gibb, R., (2011). Brain plasticity and behaviour in the developing brain. Journal Canadian Academy of Adolescent Psychiatry, 20, 265-276.

Li, Z., Tang, J., Li, H., Chen, S., He, Y., Liao, Y., ... Chen, X. (2014). Shorter telomere length in peripheral blood leukocytes is associated with childhood ASD. Scientific Reports, 47073. doi:10.1038/srep07073.

Manzoni, G., Pagnini, F., Castelnuovo, G., & Molinari, E. (2008). Relaxation training for anxiety: a ten-years systematic review with meta-analysis. Bio Med Central Psychiatry, doi:10.1186/1471-244X-8-41.

McEwen, B.S., and Morrison, J.H., (2013). The brain on stress: vulnerability and plasticity of the prefrontal cortex over the life course. Neuron, 79, 16-29.

Mosconi, M., Cody-Hazlett, H. Poe, M., Gerig, G., Gimpel-Smith, R., and Piven, J., (2009). Longitudinal study of amygdala volume and joint attention in 2- to 4-year-old children with ASD. Archives of General Psychiatry, 66, 509-516.

Radley, J.J., Rocher, A.B., Hof, P.R., McEwen, B.S., Morrison, J.H., (2005). Reversibility of apical dendritic retraction in the rat medial prefrontal cortex following repeated stress. Experimental Neurology, 196, 199-203.

Rogers, C.E., Larkey, L.K., & Keller, C. (2009). A review of clinical trials of tai chi and qigong in older adults. Western Journal of Nursing Research, 31(2), 245-279.

Schutte, N & Malouff, J. (2014). A meta-analytic review of the effects of mindfulness meditation on telomerase activity. Psychoneuroendocrinology, 42(45-48) doi: 10:1016/j.psyneuen.2013.12.017.

Tang, Y.Y., Ma, Y., Wang, J., Fan, Y., Feng, S., Lu, Q., ... Posner, M. (2007). Short-term meditation training improves attention and self-regulation. Proceedings of the National Academy of Science USA,104(43), 17152-17156.

CHAPTER 16 - TREATMENT MODEL

Karasak, R. (1979). Job demands, job decision latitude, and mental strain: implications for job redesign. Administrative Science Quarterly Vol. 24, No. 2, pp. 285-308.

Sherman, G., Lee, J., Cuddy, A., Renshon, J., Oveis, C., Gross, J., & Lerner, J. (2012) Leadership is associated with lower levels of stress. PNAS October 30, 2012 109 (44) 17903-17907; https://doi.org/10.1073/pnas.1207042109.

CHAPTER 17 - MINIMIZING STRESSORS

Alcañiz Raya M, Chicchi Giglioli IA, Marín-Morales J, Higuera-Trujillo JL, Olmos E, Minissi ME, Teruel Garcia G, Sirera M and Abad L (2020) Application of Supervised Machine Learning for Behavioral Biomarkers of Autism Spectrum Disorder Based on

Electrodermal Activity and Virtual Reality. Front. Hum. Neuroscience 14:90. doi: 10.3389/fnhum.2020.00090.

CHAPTER 18 - PROMOTING RELAXATION

Tang, Y.Y., Ma, Y., Wang, J., Fan, Y., Feng, S., Lu, Q., ... Posner, M. (2007). Short-term meditation training improves attention and self-regulation. Proceedings of the National Academy of Science USA,104(43), 17152-17156.

CHAPTER 19 - TREATING STRESS DURING PREGNANCY

Alda, M., Puebla-Guedea, M., Rodero, B., Demarzo, M., Montero-Marin, J., Roca, M., & Garcia-Campayo, J., (2016). Zen meditation, Length of Telomeres, and the Role of Experiential Avoidance and Compassion. Mindfulness, 7:651-659, DOI:10.1007/s12671-016-0500-5.

Buss, C., Davis, E.P., Muftuler, T., Head, K., & Sandman, C., (2010). High pregnancy anxiety during mid-gestation is associated with decreased gray matter density in 6-9-year-old children. Psychoneuroendicrinology 35,141-153.

Cheslack-Postava, K., Liu, K & Bearman, P. (2011). Closely spaced pregnancies are associated with increased odds of autism in California sibling births. Pediatrics, 127(2) 246-253.

DiPietro, J.A., Costigan, K.A., Nelson, P., Gurewitsch, E.D. & Laudenslager, M.L. (2008). Fetal responses to induced maternal relaxation during pregnancy. [Abstract] Biological Psychiatry, 77(1), 11-19.

Epel, E., Blackburn, E., Lin, J., Dhabhar, F., Adler, N., Morrow, J., & Cawthon, R., (2004). Accelerated telomere shortening in response to life stress. PNAS, doi:10.1073.

Heinrichs, M., Baumgartner, T., Kirschbaum, C., and Ehlert, U., (2003). Social support and oxytocin interact to suppress cortisol and subjective responses to psychosocial stress. Society of Biological Psychiatry, 54, 1389-1398.

Ram, S., Howland, M., Sandman, C., Davis, E., & Glynn, L. (2018). Prenatal Risk for Autism Spectrum Disorder (ASD): Fetal Cortisol Exposure Predicts Child ASD Symptoms. Clinical Psychological Science. https://doi.org/10.1177/2167702618811079

Ronald, A., Pennell, C., & Whitehouse, A. (2011). Prenatal maternal stress associated with ADHD and autistic traits in early childhood. Frontiers in Psychology, 1(223). doi: 10.3389/fpsyg.2010.00223.

CHAPTER 20 - TREATING INFANTS

Çaka, S. & Gözen, D. (2017) Effects of swaddled and traditional tub bathing methods on crying and physiological responses of newborns. https://doi.org/10.1111/jspn.12202 J Spec Pediatr Nurs. 2018 Jan; 23(1). doi: 10.1111/jspn.12202.

Candia, M., Osaka, E., Leite, M., Toccolini, B., Costa, N., Teixeira, S. ... & Osaku, N. (2014). Influence of prone positioning on premature newborn infant stress assessed by means of salivary cortisol measurement: pilot study. Rev Bras Ter Intensiva. 26(2):169-75.

Carnes, D., Plunkett, A., Ellwood, J., & Miles, C. (2018). Manual therapy for unsettled, distressed and excessively crying infants: a systematic review and meta-analyses. BMJ Open 2018;8:e019040. doi:10.1136/ bmjopen-2017-019040.

De Bernardo, G., Riccitelli, M., Giordano, M., Proietti, F., Sordino, D., Longini, M., ... & Perrone, S.(2018). Rooming-in reduces salivary cortisol level of newborn. Mediators Inflamm. 2018 Mar 8;2018:2845352. doi:10.1155/2018/2845352.

Feldman, R., Rosenthal, A., & Eidelman, A., (2014) Maternal-preterm skin-to-skin contact enhances child physiologic organization and cognitive control across the first 10 years of life. Biological Psychiatry, 2014; 75 (1): 56 DOI: 10.1016/j.biopsych.2013.08.012.

Feldman, R., Singer, M., Zagoory, O. (2010). Touch attenuates infants' physiological reactivity to stress. Developmental Science, 13(2), 271-278.

Grunau R, Haley D., Whitfield M., Weinberg J., Yu W. & Thiessen, P. (2007). Altered basal cortisol levels at 3, 6, 8 and 18 months in infants born at extremely low gestational age. J. Pediatr. 2007;150:151–156. doi: 10.1016/j.jpeds.2006.10.053.

Hernandez-Reif, M., Diego, M., & Field, T., (2007). Preterm infants show reduced stress behaviors and activity after 5 days of massage therapy. Infant Behav Dev. 30(4): 557-561. doi: 10.1016/j.infbeh.2007.04.002.

Kurihara, H., Chiba, H., Shimizu, Y., Yanaihara, T., Takeda, M., Kawakami, K., & Takai- Kawakami, K. (1996). Behavioral and adrenocortical responses to stress in neonates and the stabilizing effects of maternal heartbeat on them. Early Hum Dev. 46(1-2):117-27. DOI: 10.1016/0378-3782(96)01749-5.

Mörelius, E., Theodorsson, E., & Nelson, N. (2015). Salivary cortisol reactivity in preterm infants in neonatal intensive care: an integrative review. International Journal of Environmental Research and Public Health, 17 Mar 2016, 13(3).

Neu, M., Zhaoxing, P., & Workman, R., Marcheggiani-Howard, Furuta, G., ...Laudenslager, M. (2013). Benefits of massage therapy for infants with symptoms of gastroesophageal reflux disease. Biological Research for Nursing Volume: 16,issue: 4, page(s): 387-397.4. https://doi.org/10.1177/1099800413516187.

Niemi, A. (2017) Review of Randomized Controlled Trials of Massage in Preterm Infants. Children (Basel). 4(4). pii: E21. doi: 10.3390/children4040021.

Provenzi, L., Fumagalli, M., Sirgiovanni, I., Giorda, R., Pozzoli, U., Morandi, F. ....

Montirosso R. (2015). Pain-related stress during the Neonatal Intensive Care Unit stay and SLC6A4 methylation in very preterm infants. Frontiers Behavioral Neuroscience. 9: 99.

Romero-Gonzales, B., Caparros-Gonzalex, R., Gonzalez-Perez, R., Delgado-Puertes, P. , Peralta- Ramirez, M. (2018). Newborn infants' hair cortisol levels reflect chronic maternal stress during pregnancy. PLoS One. 2018; 13(7): e0200279.

Schwilling, D., Vogeser, M., Kirchhoff, F., Schwaiblmair, F., Boulesteix, A., Schulze, A., ... Flemmer, A. (2015). Live music reduces stress levels in very low-birthweight infants. Acta Paediatr. 2015 Apr;104(4):360-7. doi: 10.1111/apa.12913. Epub 2015 Feb 7.

Seehagen, S., Schneider, S., Rudolph, J., Ernst, S., & Zmyj, N., (2015). Stress impairs cognitive flexibility in infants. Proceedings of the National Academy of Sciences 112 (41) 12882-12886; doi: 10.1073/pnas. 1508345112.

Silva, L., Schalock, M., Gabrielsen, K., Budden, S., Buenrostro, M., & Horton, G., (2015). Early Intervention with a Parent-Delivered Massage Protocol Directed at Tactile Abnormalities Decreases Severity of Autism and Improves Child-to-Parent Interactions: A Replication Study. Autism Research and Treatment, dos:10.1155/2015/904585.

White-Traut, R., Schwartz, D., McFarlin, B., & Kogan, J. (2009). Salivary cortisol and behavioral state responses of healthy newborn infants to tactile-only and multisensory interventions. J Obstet Gynecol Neonatal Nurs. 38(1):22-34. doi: 10.1111/j. 1552-6909.2008.00307.x.Published online 2015 Apr 21. doi: 10.3389/fnbeh.2015.00099.

CHAPTER 21 - TREATING STRESS IN CHILDREN

Brefczynski-Lewis, J.A., Lutz, A., Schaefer, H.S., Levinson, D.B., and Davidson, R.J., (2007). Neural correlates of attentional expertise in long-term meditation practitioners. PNAS, 104, 11483-11488.

Corbett, B.A., Schupp, C.W., Levine, S., & Mendoza, S. (2009). Comparing cortisol, stress, and sensory sensitivity in children with autism. Autism Research, 2(1), 39-49.

Field, T., (2014). Massage therapy research review. Complementary Therapies in Clinical Practice, 20(14), 224-229.

Kilpatrick, L.A., Suyenobu, B.Y., Smith, S.R., Bueller, J.A., Goodman, T., Creswell, J.D., ... Naliboff, B.D., (2011). Impact of mindfulness-based stress reduction training on intrinsic brain connectivity. NeuroImage, 56, 290-298.

Neece, C., (2013) Mindfulness☒Based Stress Reduction for Parents of Young Children with Developmental Delays: Implications for Parental Mental Health and Child Behavior Problems. Journal of Applied Research in Intellectual Disabilities, https://doi.org/10.1111/jar.12064.

O'Haire, M. E., McKenzie, S. J., McCune, S., & Slaughter, V. (2014). Effects of classroom animal-assisted activities on social functioning in children with autism spectrum disorder. The Journal of Alternative and Complementary Medicine, 20(3), 162-168. doi:10.1089/acm.2013.0165.

O'Haire, M. McKenzie, S., Beck, A., & Slaughter, V., (2015). Animals may act as social buffers: Skin conductance arousal in children with autism spectrum disorder in a social context. Dev Psychobiol, 57(5):584-95. doi: 10.1002/dev.21310.

Pinar, R., & Afsar, F. (2015). Back massage to decrease state anxiety, cortisol level, blood pressure, heart rate and increase sleep quality in family caregivers of patients with cancer: a randomized controlled trial. Asian Pacific Journal of Cancer Prevention: APJCP, 16(18), 8127-8133.

Pusponegoro, H., Efar, P., Soedjatmiko, Soebadi, A., Firmansyah, A., Chen, H., Hung, K. (2016). Gross motor profile and its association with socialization skills in children with Autism Spectrum Disorders. Pediatr Neonatol. 57(6):501-507. doi: 10.1016/j.pedneo. 2016.02.004. Epub 2016.

Ridderinkhof, A., de Bruin, E., Blom, R., Bogels, S. (2018). Mindfulness-based program for children with autism spectrum Disorder and their parents: direct and long-term improvements. Mindfulness (N Y). 2018;9(3):773-791. doi: 10.1007/s12671-017-0815-x.

Silva, L. & Schalock, M. (2013a). Prevalence and significance of abnormal tactile responses in young children with autism. North American Journal of Medicine and Science, 6(3), pp. 121–127.

Silva, L., & Schalock, M. (2013b). Treatment of tactile impairment in young children with autism: results with qigong massage. International Journal of Therapeutic Massage & Bodywork, vol. 6, no. 4, pp.12–20.

Silva, L., Schalock, M., Gabrielsen, K., Budden, S., Buenrostro, M., & Horton, G., (2015). Early intervention with a parent-delivered massage protocol directed at tactile abnormalities decreases severity of autism and improves child-to-parent interactions: a replication study. Autism Research and Treatment, doi:10.1155/2015/904585.

Sotoodeh, M., Arabameri, E., Panahibakhsh, M., Kheiroddin, F., Mirdoozandeh, H., Ghanizadeh, A. (2017). Effectiveness of yoga training program on the severity of autism. Complement Ther Clin Pract; 28:47-53. doi: 10.1016/j.ctcp.2017.05.001.

Wegner, M., Koutsandreou, F., Muller-Alcazar, A., Lauterbach, F., & Budde, H. (2019). Effects of different types of exercise training on the cortisol awakening response in children. Frontiers in Endocrinology, 10:463. doi: 10.3389/fendo.2019.00463.

CHAPTER 22 - PARENTS' STRESS

Abbeduto, L., Seltzer, M. & Shattuck, P. (2004) Psychological well-being and coping in mothers of youth with autism, Down Syndrome, or Fragile X Syndrome. American Journal of Mental Retardation, Vol 109, 3:237-254.

Aschbacher, K., Milush, J., Gilbert, A., Almeida, C., Sinclair, E., Epling, L., ... Epel, E. (2017). Chronic stress is associated with reduced circulating hematopoietic progenitor cell number: a maternal caregiving model. Brain Behav Immun. 2017 Jan; 59: 245–252.

Dyknes, E., Fisher, M., Taylor, J., Lambert, W., & Miodrag, N., (2014). Reducing distress in mothers of children with autism and other disabilities: a randomized trial. Pediatrics, doi:10.1542/peds.2013-3164.

Engert V, Plessow F, Miller R, Kirschbaum C, & Singer T. (2014). Cortisol increase in empathic stress is modulated by emotional closeness and observation modality. Psychoneuroendocrinology. 45:192–201. doi: 10.1016/j.psyneuen.2014.04.005.

Epel, E., Blackburn, E., Lin, J., Dhabhar, F., Adler, N., Morrow, J., & Cawthon, R., (2004). Accelerated telomere shortening in response to life stress. PNAS, doi:10.1073.

Hayes, S. & Watson, S. (2013) The impact of parenting stress: a meta-analysis of studies comparing the experience of parenting stress in parents of children with and without autism spectrum disorder. J Autism Dev Disord. 2013 Mar;43(3):629-42. doi: 10.1007/s10803-012-1604-y.

Li, Z., Tang, J., Li, H., Chen, S., He, Y., Liao, Y., ...Chen, X. (2014). Shorter telomere length in peripheral blood leukocytes is associated with childhood autism. Sci Rep. 2014; 4: 7073. doi: 10.1038/srep07073.

Nelson, C. A., Varcin, K. J., Coman, N. K., DeVivo, I., & Tager-Flusberg, H. (2015). Shortened telomeres in families with a propensity to ASD. Journal of the American Academy Of Child And Adolescent Psychiatry, 54(7), 588-594. dos:10.1016/j.jaac.2015.04.006.

Yusuf, S. Hawken, S., Ounpuu, S., Dans, T., Avezum, A. Lanas, F. ...Lisheng, L. Effect of potentially modifiable risk factors associated with myocardial infarction in 52 countries (the INTERHEART study): case-control study. Lancet. 2004 Sep 11-17;364(9438): 937-52. Published online 2016 Sep 10. doi: 10.1016/j.bbi.2016.09.009.

CHAPTER 23 - ASSESSMENT & DIAGNOSIS

Lai, T., Wright, W. & Shay, J. (2018) Comparison of telomere length measurement method Phil. Trans. R. Soc. B. http://doi.org/10.1098/rstb.2016.0451.

Ljung R, Sorqvist P, Hygge S., (2009) Effects of road traffic noise and irrelevant speech on children's reading and mathematical performance. Noise Health; 11:194-8.

McEwen, B. (2019) What is the confusion with cortisol? Chronic Stress Volume 3: 1–3 sagepub.com/journals-permissions DOI: 10.1177/2470547019833647 journals.sagepub.com/home/css.

Montpetit, A., Alhareeri, A., Montpetit, M., Starkweather, A., Elmore, L., Filler, K., ... & Jackson-Cook, C. (2014) Telomere length: a review of methods for measurement.

Nurs Res. 2014 Jul-Aug;63(4):289-99. doi: 10.1097/NNR.0000000000000037.

Raya, M., Gigliola, I., Marin-Morales, J., Higuera-Trujillo, J., Olmos, E., ...& Abad, L. (2020). Application of Supervised Machine Learning for Behavioral Biomarkers of Autism Spectrum Disorder Based on Electrodermal Activity and Virtual Reality. Frontiers of Human Neuroscience, https://doi.org/10.3389/fnhum.2020.0090.

Révész D., Milaneschi, Y., Verhoeven, J., Penninx, B. (2014). Telomere length as a marker of cellular aging is associated with prevalence and progression of metabolic syndrome. J Clin Endocrinol Metab.(12):4607-15. doi: 10.1210/jc.2014-1851.

CHAPTER 24 - PREVENTING STRESS GLOBALLY

Conner, J., Pope, D., & Galloway, M. (2009). Success with less stress. Educational Leadership | Volume 67 | Number 4 Health and Learning Pages 54-58.

Feldman, R., Singer, M., Zagoory, O. (2010). Touch attenuates infants' physiological reactivity to stress. Developmental Science, 13(2), 271-278.

Gunnar, M., Kryzer, E., Van Ryzin, M., Philips, D. (2010). The rise in cortisol in family daycare: associations with aspects of care quality, child behavior, and child sex. Child Dev. 2010 May-Jun; 81(3): 851–869. doi: 10.1111/j.1467-8624.2010.01438.x.

Hardy L. (2003). Overburdened, overwhelmed. Am. Sch. Board J. 190 18–23.

Hirvikoski, T., Mittendorfer-Rutz, E., Boman, M., Larsson, H., Lichtenstein, P., & Bölte, S. (2016). Premature mortality in autism spectrum disorder. The British Journal of Psychiatry, 1-7.doi:10.1192bjp.bp.114.160192.

Kirby, A., Bakian, A., Zhang, Y., Bilder, D., Keeshin, B., & Coon, H.(2019). A 20-year study of suicide death in a statewide autism population. Autism Research 12(4): 658-666. doi: 10.1002/aur.2076.

Martinez, T. & Zhao, Y. (2018) The impact of mindfulness training on middle grades students' office referrals. Research in Middle Level Education Vol 41, 2018 - Issue 3.

Nepon, J. Belik, S., Bolton, J.,& Serene, J. (2010). The relationship between anxiety disorders and suicide attempts: Findings from the national epidemiological survey on alcohol and related conditions. Depress Anxiety. 27(9): 791-798. DOI: 10.1002/da.20674.

O'Connor, D., Green, J., Ferguson, E., O'Carroll, R., & O'Connor, R. (2017). Cortisol reactivity and suicidal behavior: Investigating the role of hypothalamic-pituitary-adrenal axis responses to stress in suicide attempters and ideators. Psychoneuroendocrinology. 2017 Jan;75:183-191. doi: 10.1016/j.psyneuen 2016.10.019. Epub 2016 Oct 24.

Suldo, S. M., Shaunessy, E., & Hardesty, R. (2008). Relationships among stress, coping, and mental health in high-achieving high school students. Psychology in the Schools,

45(4), 273–290. https://doi.org/10.1002/pits.20300.

Van Steensel, F. J. A., Bögels, S. M., & Perrin, S. (2011). Anxiety disorders in children and adolescents with autistic spectrum disorders: A meta-analysis. Clinical Child and Family Psychology Review, 14, 302–317.

Zenner, C., Herdleben-Kurz, S. & Walach, H., (2014). Mindfulness-based interventions in schools-a systematic review and meta-analysis. Front Psychol. 2014; 5: 603.doi: 10.3389/fpsyg.2014.00603.

John Hoch - Editor
Pol Sans - Layout design
Milagros Díaz - Cover design
Heidi Scheing - Headshot

ACKNOWLEDGEMENTS

Perhaps the most challenging single page of this book is trying to thank all who assisted me throughout the ten years spent writing this book. This includes people who simply offered encouragement along the way. My gratitude to those who helped get me through. I don't mean to suggest that I ever considered quitting, but I did stumble; I did get lost; and I did get tired. These contributors picked me up, redirected me, and refreshed me:

I am grateful that my recently deceased mentor, the esteemed neuroscientist, Bruce McEwen, had faith in me.

I am appreciative that Ron Miros was willing to hold my fingers to the fire from beginning to end. He made an enormous contribution to this book.

My gratitude to the trainers who gave up their Saturday mornings to assist: Maureen Quinlan, Caitlin Kilmer, Ted Nawalinski, and David Simkins.

I also am grateful to the children and their parents who continued to show up.

I am thankful to the overburdened teachers who completed a pile of test protocols and interviews.

I was also fortunate to have the ear of my dear friend, Catherine Blansfield, who listened tirelessly to my endless hours of monologue. Catherine taught me not all daycares are alike.

Thanks to Susan Karlson who encouraged me to think some more when I just wanted to be done with it.

I was fortunate to have the assistance of those willing to dot my i's and cross my t's. These kind people assisted with clerical tasks: Bernie Weed, Sue Manning, and Valerie Hecht.

Janet Allen's keen eye assisted in proofreading. Thanks Jan.

These wonderful individuals kept me afloat. My apologies to anyone I have overlooked.

"First, a new theory is attacked as absurd, then it is admitted to be true, but obvious and insignificant; finally it is seen to be so important that its adversaries claim that they themselves discovered it."

William James

MEET THE AUTHOR ...

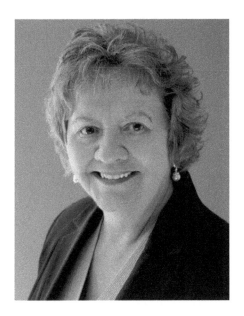

CHERYL L. NYE
PSYCHOLOGIST

Nye's pioneering research changes the face of autism. She has presented at the National Autism Conference, the International ADHD Conference, and the International Association of Behavioral Analysts. Her presentations are captivating and encourage audience participation. Nye offers staff training and program development to agencies. She currently serves as the Executive Director of the Child Stress Center. Her expertise is called upon to critique research for the Journal of Autism and Developmental Disorders.

Contact: http://childstresscenter.com

CPSIA information can be obtained
at www.ICGtesting.com
Printed in the USA
BVHW061846220222
629773BV00009B/684

9 781735 357713